TACKLING

Selective Mutism

A GUIDE FOR PROFESSIONALS AND PARENTS

Edited by Benita Rae Smith and Alice Sluckin

Foreword by Jean Gross

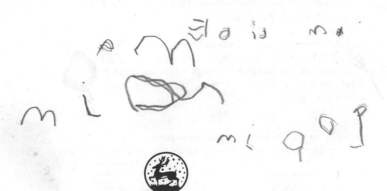

Jessica Kingsley *Publishers*
London and Philadelphia

Figures 11.1 and 11.2 on pages 176–7 reproduced with kind permission from Suffolk Learning & Improvement Service. Figure 11.3 on page 184 reproduced with kind permission from East Kent Hospitals University NHS Foundation Trust. Figure 11.4 on page 186 reproduced with kind permission from Ealing Hospital NHS Trust. Case study in Chapter 13 reproduced with kind permission from the *British Journal of Music Therapy*. All other case studies in this book have been anonymised and reproduced with the subjects' and/or guardians' permission.

First published in 2015
by Jessica Kingsley Publishers
73 Collier Street
London N1 9BE, UK
and
400 Market Street, Suite 400
Philadelphia, PA 19106, USA

Library of Congress Cataloging in Publication Data
Tackling selective mutism : a guide for professionals and
parents / edited by Benita Rae Smith and Alice
Sluckin ; foreword by Jean Gross.
    pages cm
Includes bibliographical references and index.
ISBN 978-1-84905-393-8 (alk. paper)
1. Selective mutism--Treatment. I. Smith, Benita Rae, 1934- II. Sluckin, Alice.
RJ506.M87T33 2015
618.92'855--dc23
                    2014031645

British Library Cataloguing in Publication Data
A CIP catalogue record for this book is available from the British Library

ISBN 978 1 84905 393 8
eISBN 978 0 85799 761 2

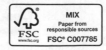

MIX
Paper from
responsible sources
FSC® C007785

Printed and bound in Great Britain by Bell and Bain Ltd, Glasgow

Dedicated to the memory of
Sylvia Baldwin, BA (Hons), MSc
who died on 12 September 2013

Sylvia was one of the first British psychologists to
understand and publish professional accounts of the needs
of children with Selective Mutism nearly 30 years ago and to
explain how they could be helped.

Contents

PART I CURRENT UNDERSTANDING OF SELECTIVE MUTISM

PART II RELATED AND CO-MORBID CONDITIONS

PART III INTERVENTIONS, STRATEGIES AND SUPPORTS

PART IV CONCLUSION

Foreword

I had my first experience of Selective Mutism (SM) or Elective Mutism, as it was then called 30 years ago. Early in my career as an educational psychologist I was asked to 'see' a little girl called Tanya who did not talk to adults in school but did whisper to a few close friends, and talked freely at home. I sat down with her in a quiet, private room and got out some blocks for her to use to copy patterns. She soon began to chat to me and over the next few weeks we were able to get her talking to teachers quite quickly, using tape recordings and the 'sliding-in' technique described in this book.

I still recall the feelings I and others had at the time. On my part I felt inordinate pride that this little girl had trusted me enough to talk to me, and satisfaction that my professional mystique as a so-called expert had been confirmed to the school's headteacher (of whom I was somewhat scared). On the part of the child's teacher, there were complicated feelings of frustration, rejection and even anger at a child who confounded reasonable everyday expectations around communication in the classroom.

In our adult lives, we often experience silence as a weapon, and communication through speech as a gift bestowed. So it was easy at that time for SM to be seen as a deliberate choice made by stubborn children. Fortunately, we have moved on from that now and are able to identify SM for what it is – a particularly disabling form of anxiety.

We have moved on in practice, too, with wider knowledge of how to treat that anxiety and enable children and young people to escape from an identity as a non-speaker in school that often entraps them for years. Much of the credit for these improvements lies with the Selective Mutism Information & Research Association (SMIRA), whose founders and supporters have worked so hard to produce this book.

It is a uniquely helpful book, representing as it does the voices of children, young people and families as well as the voices of professionals. It is full of the vivid stories of individuals, which bring home to us what it is like to experience terror on a daily basis, and the social isolation that can follow. It illustrates the power of small voluntary organizations, such as SMIRA, which bring families, carers and professionals together to share their knowledge and expertise.

The book provides remarkable historical insights: SM acts as a paradigm for developments in psychology over the past 50 years, from psychodynamic to behaviourist to ecological to cognitive behaviourist to neurolinguistic programming theories, and these are well represented in the text.

Finally, and not least, the book provides practical guidance on treatment, highlighting, for example, how advances in technology, such as being able to use a mobile device to film a child talking at home and show this in school, are radically changing approaches to early intervention.

I particularly welcome the book's very useful accounts of the way different agencies are developing agreed, shared pathways for early identification, assessment and action. This multi-agency approach seems to me the core of what is needed. SM challenges professional boundaries. Is a child not speaking because he or she is learning English as an additional language and is in the 'silent' phase? Might the silence indicate secrets that the child has been told to hide? Has the child a specific language impairment, or mental health issues? Is the classroom environment one that makes children feel comfortable?

Answering these questions requires a range of specialist expertise, variously located in educational psychology, ethnic minority achievement, child and adolescent mental health, social work and speech and language therapy services. Yet the potential for children to fall between the cracks of different services is enormous. And at a time when budgets are stretched, the temptation is for services to pass the buck, each saying that meeting speech, language and communication needs is someone else's job.

One of my major roles as the government's Communication Champion for Children between 2009 and 2011 was to meet with local commissioners in health, education and social care to communicate the effects on children of this buck-passing, and encourage them to pool budgets and commission integrated pathways of care for all children and young people with speech, language and communication needs.

We are still a long, long way from seeing that happen across the country. Where joint commissioning happens, it is likely to be only for a small minority of children with the most complex special educational needs. Yet SM tends not to fall into that category. What these children need is not an elaborate bureaucratic assessment that takes six months or more. They need a rapid response from a professional with appropriate skills, who might be an educational psychologist or a speech and language therapist, follows an agreed local pathway of care and is able to call on professionals from other backgrounds as needed, while remaining the key-worker for the family and school.

The assessment and treatment of SM, then, provides a paradigm not only for how psychology has developed but also for what we need to do for children with all kinds of speech, language and communication needs. Children suffer when we do not know what box to put them in. They need teachers, therapists, mental health professionals and social workers who work together to transcend professional boundaries, and who see parents or carers as equal partners throughout.

I should not have had to respond to that referral on my own 30 years ago. I should have been able to seek advice from a range of experts. Luckily, in a case where the difficulties were not severe or entrenched, it was possible to find solutions. But I, and more importantly Tanya, might not have been so lucky. These things are too important to leave to chance.

This book represents a major step forward in improving joined-up services for children with SM. I hope it will be read by commissioners, parents, carers and practitioners everywhere.

Jean Gross, CBE, January 2014

Acknowledgements

We are extremely grateful to the following people:

The children and families who made it possible for this book to be even considered

Dr Agnes Hauck for valuable professional guidance over a long period

Alison Huneke of the Association for All Speech Impaired Children (Afasic) for helpline advice

Annie Elias, Jane Shaw, Hilary Cleator and Professor Paul Carding for advice on functional voice disorders

Helen Webb and Denise Lanes for collaboration in the preparation of Chapter 9

Victoria Roe for meticulous fact-checking in Chapter 4

Kumi Andoh for services above and beyond mere translation from the Japanese

Lucy Buckroyd and Kate Mason, our editors at Jessica Kingsley Publishers, for unfailing support and encouragement

Our own families for tolerance, endless support, helpful comment and proofreading.

Royalties from this book will be donated to SMIRA (Selective Mutism Information & Research Association) and Afasic (Association for all Speech Impaired Children).

CHAPTER 1

Introducing Selective Mutism and an Overview of Approaches

Alice Sluckin and Rae Smith

This book was conceived as a companion volume to a fictional book published by Jessica Kingsley Publishers: *Can I tell you about Selective Mutism?* (Johnson and Wintgens 2012). This was written by two specialist speech and language therapists from the point of view of a fictional selectively mute child, and it reveals much of what children have told their helpers over the years.

The chapters of the present book have been collected in response to some of the needs of such children and their families.

Selective Mutism (SM) is a relatively rare and, until recently, little understood emotional disorder of childhood. These children converse fluently with intimates, usually in the privacy of their home, but do not speak in unfamiliar environments to people they are not familiar with, even sometimes those related to them. Much more rarely a child may speak outside the home but not within it. There is evidence in the literature (Cline and Baldwin 2004, pp.44–5) that a small minority of SM children have experienced some form of abuse or rejection in the home. Most SM children don't speak at school to their teacher or peers, but may collaborate in classroom activities non-verbally and communicate by gestures, although some of them even have difficulty making eye contact and can appear withdrawn and defensive.

In the past these children were thought to be stubborn and contrary, but more recent research indicates that the majority of them are anxious (Johnson and Wintgens 2001; Cline and Baldwin 2004), a view that official classifications now recognize.

There is speculation that, for some individuals, overwhelming anxiety may even result in temporary paralysis of the larynx, and it is beyond doubt that many who appear superficially calm are avoiding anxiety by avoiding speech.

Alice Sluckin now describes SM on the basis of her lengthy experience

As one of the editors of this book, I would like to share with you what I learned about SM while helping such children and their parents and working over many years in a clinical setting. I hope this introduction will also contribute to a better understanding of the chapters written by parents about their SM children and of those recovered sufferers in the text. Next I want to tell you more about the SM child's problem within his/her family.

Parents coping with an SM child

Parents often first notice SM when the child enters a nursery at the age of three. Since it is a relatively rare condition, thought to occur in approximately one per cent of the population (Bergman, Piacentini and McCracken 2002), misdiagnosis of separation anxiety may be made. Parents may describe some of these children as being shy and timid, but also at other times as noisy and non-compliant and also oversensitive to noise and touch, as well as unable to tolerate a change of routine. There may also be problems at bedtime.

Parents may find the child difficult to manage, particularly as they may not have come across another family with an SM child before. The family's health visitor may refer the child to the local general practitioner (GP) who hopefully might recommend referral to a speech and language therapist (SLT) and psychologist. The earlier the better, so that medical, neurological and cognitive problems can be excluded and possible co-morbidity (co-existing conditions) explored.

Unless SM is recognized early it can become entrenched, and in time will seriously interfere with the child's social, emotional and cognitive development.

What causes SM?

No single cause has been established. Research points to the presence of genetic factors (Cline and Baldwin 2004), as SM is more likely to occur if there are other members of the family showing similar behavioural traits.

A child's inborn temperament may also play a role in causation. Kagan and Snidman (2004), two internationally known researchers into biological and neurological aspects of innate childhood temperament, observed that 10–15 per cent of all newborns may be having problems with regard to adapting to unfamiliar people as well as being unable to face change. They called such children 'behaviourally inhibited to the unfamiliar'. When tested at four weeks and retested at 11 years they were more likely to be found shy and timid. It is possible that some SM children belong to this group.

There is international agreement that girls are more likely to be affected (Wright 1968; Cline and Baldwin 2004). Very bright children as well as children with learning disabilities can become selectively mute. Speech delay has been found to play a significant part in causation (Kolvin and Fundudis 1981). The condition is more frequent in ethnic minority families (Brown and Lloyd 1975; Cline and Baldwin 2004). Also, twins are more prone to SM (Wallace 1986). Frequent moves and isolated living may be factors, as well as an unsettled home background.

The SM child in the classroom

Often the SM child does not answer the register, does not read to the teacher and does not talk to peers. At mealtimes s/he does not say 'Please' or 'Thank-you' as requested by the dinner lady, and there may be problems over going to the school toilet.

Margaret Buck (1988) was one of the first teachers to draw attention to SM, and made very useful suggestions as to how such children could be helped. She pointed out that a classroom is a language environment, and she regarded talking as the pre-eminent instrument of learning. Hence the teacher who fails to establish communication with a pupil can feel inadequate and become frustrated and angry.

An example of how even a very experienced teacher might react with frustration or even despair to a non-responding child is described in the *Times* obituary (08.06.2012) of Elizabeth Manners, late Head Mistress of Felixstowe College, Suffolk. The obituary quotes Dame Elizabeth's comments on interviewing Lady Diana Spencer, later Princess of Wales, who had applied for admission to her college. The interview went as follows:

> She (Diana) just sat there with her head drooping. I said to her that, if she were to attend Felixstowe College, she would have to speak to me and I would have to see her face, but her head drooped further. There was nothing I could do.

Fortunately, many more teachers are by now able to deal confidently with SM children. Alison Hall, an experienced teacher, describes how she taught a 10-year-old boy to speak to her and read to her, though he had never spoken in school before (Hall 2008).

Diagnosing a selectively mute child

The criteria to be used for diagnosing SM children vary in different documents. However, it is widely agreed that the simple fact that a child is known to speak confidently in some situations while remaining consistently silent in others where speech is expected is sufficient for a child to be regarded/diagnosed as SM, provided that the child is not in their first term at school or in a new country in the first six months of learning a new language. More complicated diagnostic approaches are seen as potentially misleading, since the affected children differ from one another and may well have overlapping conditions, which need to be recognized and treated alongside the mutism.

More formal diagnostic recommendations include the following:

- The American Psychiatric Association's *Diagnostic and Statistical Manual (DSM-5)* (APA 2013) has once again updated its view of SM. Previously APA (1994) classified SM in the section 'Disorders Usually First Diagnosed in Infancy, Childhood, or Adolescence'. It is now classified as an Anxiety Disorder, given that the large majority of children with SM are anxious. The diagnostic criteria are largely unchanged from *DSM-IV*.

- The *ICD 10 (International Classification of Disabilities)* (WHO 1994, update due 2014). This manual is widely used in the UK. It now adopts the term 'Selective' rather than 'Elective' Mutism as previously, and categorizes it under 'Fear and Anxiety Related Disorders' in its 'Mental and Behavioural Disorders' section. The question of comorbidity and possible exclusions from the diagnosis of SM is still under discussion.

- The UK *NICE (National Institute for Health and Care Excellence) Guidelines*, constantly in the process of being updated, now include SM as an additional or associated diagnosis rather than, as previously, a variant of social anxiety disorder (2014, p.76 and p.253). A variety of alternative forms of communication are recommended for reluctant speakers (p.79 and p.242).

It is sometimes stated that children with other disorders of communication might be excluded from a diagnosis of SM. Our view is that this can be an unhelpful exclusion, as the conditions overlap. Both difficulties need to be tackled together using a team approach.

Helping children to overcome their fears and helping parents
As was said before, the problem of SM is not a new one. Joan Tough (1976), a highly respected English educationalist, when referring to children not speaking at school thought that mutism was usually due to a number of causes, but leaving the child on their own for long periods hoping that he or she would in time begin to approach and talk to others was likely to make it more difficult. In her view, the child would then adopt a role or position from which it would be increasingly difficult to escape.

It is now realized that the prognosis with regard to recovery from SM is much more promising if treatment commences at an early age, before the child acquires a non-speaking identity and is being treated as a non-speaker by peers and teachers (Johnson and Wintgens 2001; Roe 1993, 2004).

Although most children outgrow SM, sadly it can follow some into adulthood, as can be seen in the Appendix.

Until the 1950s, the treatment of SM was largely influenced by misleading psychodynamic interpretations of the condition, which blamed difficulties in the mother–child relationship, but ignored the children's inability to speak with strangers. At that time it was not understood that the child, by not speaking, was probably avoiding being devastated by feelings of anxiety.

From the 1960s onwards there was a radical shift to a new orientation in psychology toward Behaviour Modification, an approach based on the principles of learning and developed after experiments with animals. These had shown that fears and phobias were, in many cases, learned by an individual in vulnerable situations and could be unlearned (Herbert 1959; Marks 1969).

An English educational psychologist was the first to propose that SM was learned; he also noted that such children were very anxious (Reed 1963). To understand the condition better, parents were encouraged to keep records of the child's frequency of talking to specific people in specific situations. Nor was the condition any longer perceived as primarily controlled by the affected child, but was one that was strongly influenced by the response of others. Thus Cunningham *et al.* (1983) observed that, in response to children's silence, teachers often adopt a pattern of verbal interaction (for instance, questioning) which reinforces their silence, while peers in contrast ignore them. Hence it was realized that parents and teachers were key people in the management and treatment of SM. The use of behaviour modification strategies in the treatment of SM became even more accepted after the seminal paper by Black and Uhde (1995). Thirty SM children ranging in age from 5 to 16 were studied, and it was found that their characteristics resembled children suffering from a social phobia and avoidance disorders.

When devising a behavioural programme, achievable intermediate targets must be set to enable the child by *very small* steps to move through non-verbal communication to speech, as the child's level of anxiety gradually decreases. If necessary, a behavioural approach can be combined with the use of puppets, play and music therapy, or 'cognitive-behavioural' guidance in the case of older children.

Behavioural strategies that are particularly successful in counteracting anxiety are *fading* and *shaping*:

- *Fading*, colloquially known as 'sliding-in', is used as a starting point in a situation when the child is relaxed and talking to a familiar person, usually a parent. Another person then enters the room but stays at a distance. Gradually, step by step, the new person moves nearer. Depending on the child's reaction, this can take a long time or desensitization can come about quickly. Once the new person is accepted by the child s/he becomes the main helper and the parent is faded out.

- *Shaping* consists of rewarding any sound s/he might be making by mouth such as blowing bubbles and windmills, or imitating animal noises. This is attempted if during a programme a child remains totally silent, in the hope that it will gradually lead to speech. Also, to reduce crippling anxiety, the child is taught slow breathing as well as muscle relaxation (Kearney 2010). Rewards may increase motivation.

School-based behavioural programmes, which rely on 'small steps' and gradual exposure of the child to anxiety-provoking situations, have proved very successful (Johnson and Wintgens 2001). Their starting point is when a parent is talking freely to the child in the classroom, another person, who subsequently becomes the key-person, is faded in step by step depending on when the child becomes willing to co-operate with the new person. The programme requires full parental co-operation and a key-worker, who works with the child 4–5 times a week at school for at least one term (Johnson and Wintgens 2001).

Final comments on helping parents and the SM child

Showing empathy to the family and child is crucial (Sluckin and Jehu 1969). For a helper it may be preferable to meet them initially in their home, where both parents and child are likely to be less anxious. The family may also have other problems, monetary or marital, and these should be acknowledged and advice given as to who might be able to assist. If the child is also being seen by another professional, there should be parental co-operation facilitated perhaps by the school nurse (Sluckin 2011) or Special Educational Needs Co-ordinator (SENCO).

There should be a close working relationship between the parents and the school. It is often helpful if one of the parents can spend some time each week at the child's school, perhaps working on a project suggested by the teacher, possibly in a room adjoining the classroom. Once the SM child has started to talk there, another child can join them, as this might 'break the habit of a lifetime'.

Prior to starting a programme it is important to make a warm, trusting relationship with the SM child and convey that s/he will be accepted whether s/he speaks or remains silent. Suitable toys in the playroom such as puppets, water or 'sand-world' with small figures will create the right sort of atmosphere. If the child cherishes a pet, interest should be shown in it. Pets such as cats and horses have been reported to help a child overcome reluctance to speak, and we shall re-visit this theme in Chapter 10.

Theories of anxiety development in children (Wood *et al.* 2003) suggest that children's family relationships and the type of interaction that is modelled at home can be associated with the onset of anxiety, but that the causes and sequence of the condition are complex and elusive. However, one could refer to the following and design treatment accordingly:

- predisposing factors which may be predominantly genetic

- precipitating factors located in the child's environment which may act as a trigger

- perpetuating factors which relate to the way the problem is being handled in the here and now by the parents as well as the school (Johnson and Wintgens 2001).

Fortunately, there are now, in addition to Johnson and Wintgens (2001), other useful books available on how to help the SM child, giving specific information to parents and teachers. These include Bergman (2013); Davis (2013); Kearney (2010); McHolm, Cunningham and Vanier (2005); Perednik (2013) and Rapee *et al.* (2008).

Who can help?

You will see from this book that the person helping the SM child may be a professional or a volunteer, such as a member of our charity SMIRA (see Chapter 4). Our experience is that parents are now playing an increasing role in helping one another. However, SMIRA has always taken the view that seriously affected children may need special attention and should be referred to professionals for full investigation and treatment. This is particularly vital when other conditions co-exist.

With regard to predicting recovery, it is impossible to be accurate. but the older the child is at the time of starting a programme, the more likely it is that parents will be in for a long haul!

Rae Smith continues the introduction from another point of view

Speech and language therapists (SLTs) are now asked more frequently to be part of teams tackling SM. They have special contributions to make as they are used to empathizing with speech-impaired clients, facilitating communication in challenging circumstances and identifying speech, language and communication needs (SLCN). Also, SLTs are likely to be adaptable enough to incorporate suggestion and objects of reference into treatment and to assess SM children at home if they fail to speak in schools or clinics (see Chapter 5).

However, when I worked as an SLT I was used to working with children who were completely unable to speak, or to speak intelligibly (Duffy 2005; Smith 2004; Wiesmer 2007), and this led me to feel unsympathetic to SM children. I saw them as contrary and unappreciative of the gift of speech. Also, I had been trained to think that the condition was probably intractable and that treatment should be left to psychiatrists (Smith 2004). It was only through listening to Alice and gaining access to the type of information that is presented in this book that my views changed.

How to use the book

The various chapters have been put together for the benefit of all those whose lives are touched by SM, and it will quickly become obvious that different sections will be of special relevance to different types of reader.

Chapter 2: Tony Cline's update is likely to interest everyone because of its breadth of view and because he has been one of the foremost experts in the field of SM for many years.

Chapter 3: This chapter presents an important piece of questionnaire-based research, and begins with a section that is primarily intended for fellow researchers. Readers whose interest is more personal will enjoy the chapter more if they begin at a later stage, when the 'voices' of families where SM has been a problem begin to be heard. The author is Deputy Chair of SMIRA.

Chapter 4: Anyone with an interest in how support groups are set up, used and developed will want to read this account.

Chapter 5: Co-morbidity means co-existence of various medical conditions. We hope that researchers will find this chapter to be of value. The author is a specialist speech and language pathologist whose colleagues will notice a very useful section on assessment. One of the main messages is that a person who has other communication difficulties may also have SM. Diagnostic exclusions are unhelpful, other than in making insurance-based decisions about professional responsibility.

Chapter 6: Anyone interested in the complex issue of autistic spectrum disorders will value this chapter, which has been written by a specialist SLT.

Chapter 7: This chapter explores the question of whether, or not, SM is related to stammering.

Chapter 8: This chapter is primarily the story of a young man's recovery from SM, written by a language specialist. Since medication had a part to play in this story, we were interested in dealing with the commonly asked question, 'Is it useful or best avoided?' Fortunately, an experienced child psychiatrist agreed to add a comment and a more general further section.

Chapter 9: This chapter provides accounts of how SM has been tackled in schools and beyond by various means. The descriptions are provided by professionals from a variety of disciplines.

Chapter 10: This chapter is written mostly by parents who explain exactly what they did to support their children's recovery from SM.

Chapter 11: This chapter describes the local arrangements for supporting people with SM in some areas of the UK, which we know will interest administrators and commissioners. International consensus recommendations formed the basis of these 'care pathways'.

Chapter 12: As its title suggests, this chapter contains a small selection of approaches to SM outside the UK.

Chapter 13: This chapter shows how a music therapy researcher successfully worked with an SM child. Treatment sessions and the theoretical background are described.

Chapter 14: A general issue that pervades all thinking about SM is that of speakers' confidence. Rosemary Sage has, for many years, been providing and writing about COGs (Communication Opportunity Groups). These have proved helpful to such a wide variety of young people that we were keen to include her insights.

Chapter 15: Written with an education expert, this chapter provides legal and administrative information, which should be useful to people determined to give a fair deal to SM children within the education system and outside it.

Chapter 16: This chapter allows two well-functioning young adults to describe their experience of SM, followed by their paths to recovery.

Chapter 17: Alice and Rae look back at the preparation of the book and at what they have learnt about SM over the years. They also make some recommendations.

The Appendix deals briefly with SM in adults.

People suffering from SM are individuals

Some people think of SM as rather similar to 'stage fright' in which competent individuals become nervous about speaking before the public. However, we know that actors usually recover the power of speech once the curtain has risen and it is only rarely that this sort of 'fright' prevents them from taking the stage at all. Most of the people who are situationally/selectively mute genuinely find themselves unable or compulsively reluctant to speak in certain settings.

Individuals suffering from SM can differ from one another and may be experiencing differing symptoms, motivation and emotions. A small minority are angry young people who refuse to speak as a form of protest; another minority group have experienced physical or psychological trauma; some are subject to a strong impression of taboo, or are fearful of disclosing dangerous information. Some experience other people, including peers, as hostile and react accordingly. It is now recognized that most would genuinely prefer to interact normally, but some even describe themselves as 'frozen' or unable to activate their voice.

Some find even deliberate non-verbal signalling beyond their ability when in a state of terror, but others can achieve communication non-verbally – for instance, through drawing (Miller 2008) and by carrying short messages on cards or miniature recording devices.

It is also important to understand, as Alice has pointed out, that some individuals do indeed remain silent, having learnt that talking is likely to make them feel painfully anxious, but it is by no means certain that they have made this decision consciously. Negative strategies such as this may simply provide intuitive solutions to communication difficulties. Katz-Bernstein (2013, p.25) describes several possible methods of categorizing SM and also points out that a compulsion to avoid speaking can hardly be described as a free choice. It may not be necessary to bring the question of unconscious choice to children's attention, but awareness of the role of avoidance is a vital insight for their helpers.

Approaches to these differing individuals need to be based on real relationships with the children and their families and, sometimes, on sensitive interpretation of such things as posture, face colour, frowns, sighs or averted eyes, which are truthfully communicative precisely because they are not under voluntary control

One of the challenges for teachers and therapists is that only by honestly acknowledging and examining our own responses can we can begin to guess how silent children might be reached and understood. Unfortunately, one's own reaction can be quite shaming. As professionals who claim to be positive and constructive in our relationships, we can feel surprisingly cross when children remain 'rudely' silent and evasive. A feeling of hurt and rejection is natural in the circumstances, but if this is coupled with a feeling that our professional skills are being made to appear useless, or that we are being disrespected, anger can become part of the mix. Speaking hastily while in this frame of mind to someone who already finds us alarming can only make matters worse. A more constructive response is to muse out loud in an empathetic way, rather than continuing to question a non-responsive child (see box on next page).

'It seems to me that you may be feeling a bit uncomfortable. You don't need to talk to me until we get used to one another. We can take our time. You might like to look at what the class is going to study this morning. I'll just take the register first and mark you present for today. Tomorrow, if you feel ready, we can work out a signal that you can give me.'

Why does SM matter?

First, SM is not age-appropriate behaviour and it can interfere with learning, being included in the peer group and making friends. It can also be very worrying to parents and concerned family members, especially if a child appears to be rude to people such as grandparents. It is true that sociability and quietness are valued differently by different cultural groups and that there can even be advantages to being reserved and being quiet – one gets more work done, for instance – but cutting oneself off from others entirely is not all that enjoyable. It's a matter of degree.

Gaining experience of making friends, falling out, repairing misunderstandings and so forth helps us to understand how to conduct adult relationships.

Also, there is the question of unpopularity. From time immemorial, casting individuals out of the tribe has been a serious punishment and such phrases as 'I'm not talking to you anymore' have signalled rejection and disapproval. This is why people get upset by not being spoken to. If children cannot help being silent, they may need support in coping with other people becoming hostile toward them. It is hard to miss out on the joy of friendships and to be left out of the jokes and plans made by your peer group.

From the point of view of educators, an uncommunicative child can be difficult to assess and to include in class activities. We know of individuals who have been held back inappropriately because of failure to demonstrate their abilities. In another area, Public Health England (PHE) has recognized that engaging poor communicators in public health initiatives such as alcohol awareness or prevention of teenage pregnancies can be particularly awkward.

There is also the question of acquiring social skills. Withdrawing from the arena within which these are gradually put to the test can leave one seriously short of experience. Evidence from parents and people who have recovered from SM suggests that a characteristic of some SM children is difficulty in adapting their style of interaction to unfamiliar situations, where different rules and expectations apply and a different type of understanding is required. Remaining silent when you are uncertain how to behave may well provide an opportunity to weigh things up through observation, but it clearly prevents one from practising the subtle arts of interacting and forming relationships. Any child in this position requires help, but those who also suffer from social communication disorders, sometimes known as 'pragmatic language impairment', urgently need specialized attention (Adams 2008).

Pragmatics, that is to say the use and interpretation of language in real contexts, can be an area of difficulty for teenagers who have spent even a part of their school life talking only in comfortable home situations. This is because gaining the ability to handle both the formality of classroom language and the subtle demands of informal social negotiation with peers depends upon experimentation, feedback, trial and error.

Teenage girls, in particular, can get into serious difficulties if they are not able to discern the intention behind what is said to them by boys and men or to make their own feelings and wishes clear.

Young people who have an acceptable appearance and behave in an acceptable manner with peers are not likely to face too much rejection. However, barriers to social inclusion can appear once they begin to speak. A person who has not had sufficient opportunity to practise may have poor timing. They may have difficulty in spotting transition points in conversation, judging whether interruption is possible or estimating how long a turn to take. One has to learn from experience and feedback when to relinquish the floor, when to give ground and when to stand firm, when to be formal and when a casual tone is appropriate. There are skills involved in holding topics appropriately, digressing and returning to a theme, remaining coherent, joking and indicating seriousness. Many factors in addition to the actual words chosen are involved in successful negotiation with other human beings (Cummings 2009; Leinonen *et al.* 2000; Smith and Leinonen 1992).

Teenagers, for instance, acquire a particular sensitivity to fashions, subtle messages and implications. They value the nuances of slang, 'bad language', humour, irony and wit. They pretend misunderstanding to suit their own purposes, they play with language and they always rely upon intonation or non-verbal signals to carry parts of their message. When these skills are weak, relationships with both peers and teachers suffer.

Adams has pointed out (2005, p.182) that at least four aspects of child development play a part in social communication. These are: social cognition (knowledge); verbal and non-verbal pragmatics (behaviour); receptive and expressive language processing; and 'social interaction' (experimentation and experience). Ideally, these factors influence one another as children mature and integrate what they have learnt. However, we have the impression that, if social interaction is limited for whatever reason, an individual's social skills may not develop sufficient flexibility to adapt to the variety of demands encountered in social life or in the adult working environment. It is possible for a silent person to form an impression of how social relationships work by means of observation, but it takes practice to make them work oneself.

For all these reasons, we suggest that SM cannot simply be ignored. This book was written to address some of the issues raised by Situational/Selective Mutism. However, we do not address full mutism, which is the inability to communicate in any setting, having once begun to do so (Lebrun 1990; Magagna 2013) or difficulties in developing any intelligible speech and language at all (Bercow 2008; Bishop 2008; Danon-Boileau 2001; Duffy 2005; Wiesmer 2007). These are different and more severe disorders.

PART I

Current Understanding of Selective Mutism

CHAPTER 2

Selective Mutism in Children
Changing Perspectives Over Half a Century

Tony Cline

Defining the phenomenon

In this chapter, in order to provide a context for the book, I will review how perspectives on Selective Mutism (SM) have changed over the last 50 years. It is a puzzling and unexpected pattern of behaviour. How have professionals and researchers described it and explained it over the years? How have changes in society and changes in the way we think about childhood and mental health and social development affected how we think about SM?

The main characteristics associated with SM appear simple. Here is how a mother, Sharon Longo, describes her son Brian in the Personal Stories section of the Anxiety Disorders Association of America website. Her article, which is called 'My Silent Child', begins: 'My 5-year-old boy has a cherub's face with a hint of mischief in his beautiful green eyes. Brian dances to silly music and entertains us with his antics. He tells his brother to leave him alone and he teases his sister while she does her homework. The only difference between Brian and most other children is that while he is at school, he is mute.'

Selectively mute children talk readily in some situations but not in others. The characteristics associated with this challenging pattern of behaviour may include:

- social anxiety and social phobia (fearfulness)

- physical symptoms of anxiety

- shy or sad or socially withdrawn demeanour

- oppositional, contrary, manipulative or wilful behaviour

- problems of development of communication (e.g. speech problems)

- concern (which may not be expressed openly) about the negative consequences of speaking (e.g. displaying inefficient or underdeveloped speaking skills)

- skilled compensatory behaviour (e.g. effective non-verbal communication skills)

- successful creation of an environment in which others accept and compensate for the child's silence.

(Adapted from Kearney 2010, Table 1.3)

Of course, any individual child will show only some of these features. No one will show them all.

How we name a phenomenon reflects what we think it is, and the name may also be influenced by what we think causes it. The terms used to refer to SM have changed over the years for that reason. The earliest term, 'aphasia voluntaria', was coined by the German physician Adolph Kussmaul in 1877. The Latin means 'voluntary lack of speech'. The phrase 'elective mutism' was coined in 1934 by a Swiss child psychiatrist, Moritz Tramer. He thought there was an element of choice in his patient's selection of who he would and would not talk to, even if the basis of that choice was unconscious. There appears to have been no single author who was the first to explain the addition of a letter to the beginning of 'elective' to create the term 'Selective Mutism'. Between 1967 and 1976 several groups of authors in different areas of the USA, starting with John Reid and his colleagues in Oregon (Reid *et al.* 1967), began to use the new term in the papers that they published. There was no published explanation at the time, but others took up the term and it was decisively adopted by the American Psychiatric Association in 1994. In contrast to the phrases used previously, these words seemed 'to capture the key features of the phenomenon most clearly: it is selective and it involves a lack of speech where speech is normally found. A particular advantage of this term is that it does not introduce any untested assumptions into the labelling of the behaviour. For example, it does not imply that children elect or choose to remain silent, and it does not automatically associate their pattern of behaviour with a phobic reaction' (Cline and Baldwin 2004, p.13).

Does SM express some kind of fear or phobia? As early as 1971 a multi-disciplinary team working in Rochester, New York State, used the term 'speech phobia' to refer to it (Halpern *et al.* 1971). This term has not been taken up by others, but the notion that SM may involve some form of phobia has attracted increasing attention. For example, Heidi Omdal of Stavanger in Norway has recently argued that it is best understood as 'a specific phobia of expressive speech' (Omdal and Galloway 2008). But perhaps the phobia is not so specific? A more influential idea has been that SM may be a specific symptom of a more general social phobia. In one of the first larger-scale studies of SM, Black and Uhde (1992) reported high levels of social anxiety in a sample of 30 children with SM and argued that it 'may be a symptom of social anxiety rather than a distinct diagnostic syndrome' (p.847).

An alternative perspective has been presented by a Canadian psychologist, Norman Hadley. He pointed out that the literature on SM tends to focus on uses and habits of speech. He emphasized the role that silence plays in human communication and was critical of clinicians and researchers who ignored the context of the day-to-day use of silence when treating or studying SM. 'There are many "sounds of silence" which are a part of day-to-day communication. Elective mutism is only one silence-related communication problem' (Hadley 1994, p.xxi). So he called children who are selectively mute 'silence users'. This usage is analogous to calling those whose physical movements are restricted 'wheelchair users'. It will be seen that such terms are influenced by the late twentieth-century interest in patients and people with disabilities as agents who have (or should have) control over their lives and who are (or should be) active agents in the management of the challenges they face. In some ways the argument for this shift in terminology represents a return to the emphasis on the voluntary or elective nature of the behaviour that characterized the earliest professional accounts of it, but there is a crucial change of perspective: the element of blame has been removed.

The transition from home to school

SM is usually first observed when a child starts at school or nursery. In western societies the contexts of child development up to that point have changed in many ways since the 1960s. The technology of everyday life has been transformed, of course, including the technologies of communication. There has been a shift in buying habits from small, local, family-run shops to large, area-based, impersonal supermarkets and stores. An increasing proportion of purchases are made online. As we move about the cities where most of us live, we use our individual cars much more, and when we go on a bus, we buy a ticket from a machine rather than a conductor. My colleague Sylvia Baldwin has pointed out that the effect of each shift has been that young children are less engaged in family routines that socialize them into confident everyday communication with comparative strangers. There is less communication about everyday transactions with familiar adults who are outside the family circle.

Alongside that important change in children's pre-school experience there have been developments in their exposure to institutional environments outside the home. An increasing number of children in the UK are now entering their first educational setting at around their third birthday, a stage when many are not yet confident speakers, especially to people outside the home. Nursery staff report that many children speak very little in nursery at first and that it is not uncommon for them to take a term to start talking in a relaxed way with adults. It should be noted that the age of most selectively mute children at referral for help is closely related to the time of starting school. There are no published data on the incidence of SM in nurseries and playgroups. Relatively few referrals are recorded in the literature, but they are not unknown (e.g. Tittnich 1990). At any rate, expectations appear to shift as children approach school age.

Some leeway is allowed to a pre-school child. Parents will apologize for a young child who fails to respond to an approach from another adult: 'He's not himself today.' Sylvia Baldwin observed that popular idiom has other similar let-out phrases, such as 'Has the cat got your tongue then?' This is not only a defence of the child but a face-saver for the adult who has been rebuffed. Starting school finally takes children away during the day from the group of people with whom they have had most practice in talking. For some, the challenge of separation from their mother and the familiar setting of the home is overwhelming. Most adapt to the new context, but some take a long time to do so.

In the past it was not uncommon for children in remote rural areas to experience many problems on school entry. One region where these were found at one point to include SM was Eastern Kentucky in the USA. The area concerned was in a remote region of the Appalachian Mountains. There were barriers to East–West travel that had affected the area during its colonial history. Even today there are many tiny, isolated communities. In the 1960s a new project brought 'field clinics' for children with emotional and behavioural problems to an area of Eastern Kentucky. Analyzing project records, Looff (1971) found a higher number of selectively mute children than expected (2.8% of the clinics' case load), and he suspected that there were many more who had not been referred. There was therefore a higher prevalence in that region than anywhere else in the USA. He argued that one factor contributing to this phenomenon was a generally low level of verbal communication among many families in the area. There were both silent individuals, known locally as 'quiet turned', and silent families where active practical skills were valued more than talk. This was especially true of the men, who, as Looff points out, would be trained from an early age to keep quiet while hunting or fishing.

Obviously, this strong local cultural tradition had a significant influence, but he identified a second important factor relating to the way schools were organized. An acute problem arose for some children when tiny schools with one, two or three rooms in isolated communities were closed and new 'consolidated elementary schools' were opened to cater for more than 300 pupils in a whole district. Many children were unused to travelling outside their immediate community. For some, the experience was overwhelming: 'In the classroom they remained frozen in their seats, would not say a word, and refused to move to go to the bathroom, lunchroom or playground. A few sobbed quietly as they sat. Several furtively nibbled at lunches brought from home, ceasing when noticed. None attempted to read or write' (Looff 1971, pp.80–81). According to previous school reports all these children had been considered extreme social isolates by their neighbours, but had been able to function in their former schools. The children's withdrawal, which persisted for two or three months, seemed to be an attempt to cope with the overwhelming anxiety of the unfamiliar situation.

Today in the western world the main factors in the isolation of such families are likely to be psychological, cultural and linguistic rather than physical or geographical. The incidence of SM is greater in children from ethnic and linguistic minorities. SM has been reported more frequently in the recent past in towns and cities. Schools may now face particular challenges in their role as a focus for communal socialization in atomized urban communities, just as they have done in the past in scattered rural communities. One perspective that has had some influence at intervals over the last 50 years has been a systemic approach to understanding SM, a view that it is not produced by factors within an individual or a family alone, but also by the ways that families interact with the society around them and the ways that society facilitates or inhibits that interaction.

The conditions for learning at school

It was already true of many classrooms in the 1960s that the process of learning was based, in part, on group work, shared tasks, social interaction and pooled effort. However, as long as the central goals of the school curriculum were defined in terms of the skills children needed for written examinations, a selectively mute child could get by without taking full advantage of learning strategies that relied on talking and negotiating with a peer group and active collaboration. Thus, writing in 1965, a psychiatric team working in Detroit described a selectively mute seven-year-old girl who 'did her written work (at school) exceptionally well but refused to read aloud or recite... The teacher reported that she appeared aware of her environment and liked to participate in activities. She actually did communicate by shaking or nodding her head. Because of this non-verbal communication ability, albeit limited, she had not failed in school' (Elson *et al.* 1965, p.183).

A few years later a similar team in Seattle reported on a six-year-old girl who they called Emma: 'Although she lived just across the street from the school and played actively there, she had only to cross the street to become a pliable mannequin. In addition to not speaking, Emma never participated in any motor activities. She carried home the school craft materials, and made at home the things that the others had made in class. She eagerly related to her mother all that went on in school each day and was apparently quite attentive' (Wulbert *et al.* 1973). At their university clinic, they tested Emma by observing through a one-way screen while her parents gave her their tests. They found that her intelligence was average, she knew the alphabet, could read several words, including the names of all the members of her family, and could count and write numbers to 100.

Now, however, silent achievement of traditional school skills is not enough. One of the things that has changed since the 1960s is that a social dimension is now a central feature of the school curriculum. Children must not only read and write but also speak. They must learn to work in small co-operative groups and to report back on their group discussions and their own individual work to a whole class. Assessment in school now takes account of these goals. It is no longer enough at any age to be a silent achiever. A full education for selectively mute children, as for all children, ultimately involves working towards relaxed and confident speech in the classroom.

Assessment of SM

Reading accounts of professional work and research with SM in the 1960s and 1970s, it is striking for a reader today to see the casual and unsystematic ways in which children's use of speech in different contexts was described and evaluated. A major change over the last 50 years has been the development of simple strategies for recording patterns of speaking and measuring change. Table 2.1 shows a 'Summary Grid' that Sylvia Baldwin and I developed some years ago (Cline and Baldwin 2004). An approach to this task that is visually more interesting but does not record quite so much information, the 'Talking Map', was developed by Johnson and Wintgens (2001, pp.71–73). An advantage of that approach is that children themselves can be given a copy of the 'map' and record their own habits of speech. An instrument that facilitates a similarly broad and systematic profile of a child's communication behaviour may be found in Kearney (2010).

In Table 2.1, community settings will be local places outside the home such as a park or a corner shop. It may be important to include more than one school setting so that a record can be made of a child's use of speech in their main classroom, a more intimate support room and the relatively adult-free playground. It is intended that the grid be used flexibly. Additional columns and rows can be inserted to allow for the recording of communication with a person or in a setting that is of interest in a particular case. For example, a row might have been allocated to a child's pet dog if that is the only individual or one of few who hears the child's voice regularly. A simple notation can be used to summarize whether a child speaks normally to someone or replies to questions and conversational initiatives from them but does not speak spontaneously on their own initiative, or communicates with this person in this setting only non-verbally – for example, through pointing, nodding or shaking head or other gestures. Frequency of speech and volume can also be recorded. That may be of particular interest where a child communicates with some people only in whispers.

TABLE 2.1 SUMMARY OF A CHILD'S HABITS OF SPEECH ACROSS SETTINGS

Child's name	Own home	Relative's home	Community setting 1	Community setting 2	School setting 1	School setting 2
Date						
Mother						
Father						
Sibling 1 >>						

Sibling 2 >>					
Relative 1 >>					
Relative 2 >>					
Teacher >>					
>>					
>>					

The development of SM

It has become increasingly clear that a full understanding of
SM requires a sophisticated understanding of anxiety. Most
selectively mute children show signs of a high level of anxiety about
communication, if not about other things too. Because some of the
children can be wilful, defiant and controlling as well, it was suggested
in the past that the determination and oppositional behaviour were of
central importance (e.g. Wright 1968), but in recent years it has been
increasingly recognized that – while many factors may play a part in
the development of SM – anxiety seems to be the crucial factor. It
is now commonly argued that, when the children are manipulative
or controlling in their behaviour, 'it is more helpful and accurate to
view the mutism as an involuntary defence against the child's severe
anxiety' (Anstendig 1999, p.429). The overall picture was possibly
concealed in the past because most studies of children with SM were
based on individual clinic cases, in which the descriptions of defiant
and wilful children were very striking. When survey methods began
to be used to study larger numbers of selectively mute children, it
became clear that the majority were shy and anxious rather than
oppositional or negative. This has been confirmed in a series of area
surveys and follow-up studies starting in the 1990s (e.g. Black and
Uhde 1995; Steinhausen and Juzi 1996).

The view that anxiety is a central factor in SM has been further
strengthened by the observation that some selectively mute children
are rather inactive and passive, which is seen as suggestive of an
underlying heightened level of anxiety. If genetic propensity plays a
role in SM, it may be relevant that other family members are often
reported to appear shy and anxious too. It is significant that those
children who have associated problems, in addition to their mutism,
tend to present with anxiety-related problems such as social phobia
rather than motivational or conduct problems. But why do a small
proportion of the children who have difficulties with anxiety focus
their concerns on communication and remain silent in the presence
of some of those they meet? It is not enough to understand that
SM may have its roots in anxiety; we need to go further to identify
how anxiety which is expressed in many different behaviours by

other children finds a very unusual form of expression in this group. Table 2.2 (page 46) reproduces an account of the process that Sylvia Baldwin and I developed some time ago (Cline and Baldwin 2004, Table 3.3).

One aim of this account is to make clear that, as the example from the Appalachian Mountains above illustrated, factors in the community as well as factors in the child and the family may play a part in the process. Adopting a traditional behavioural framework, this figure differentiates between disposing factors that create a situation that is favourable to the development of SM, precipitating factors that trigger the behaviour on the first few occasions, and maintaining factors that keep it going. It is not necessary to have factors operating at each of the levels (the community, the family and the child) for full-blown SM to develop, but when there are active influences at more than one level we can anticipate that that will be more likely – a hypothesis that has not been tested through systematic research.

There has been a shift in research attention over the past 50 years. Up to and during the 1960s a great deal of emphasis was placed on the risk factors within the family. From the 1970s and into the early 1980s ecological factors outside the family are mentioned much more often. At the same time, during the 1970s an interest in learning theory and behaviour therapy led to a greater emphasis on the factors that keep SM going – reinforcement from other people's reaction to the child's communication profile (family members and others). Steadily, in recent years, advances in genetics have led to increasing interest in the possibility that children who are selectively mute have a temperamental predisposition to SM. Finally, during the last 20 years increasing attention has been paid to the argument that many factors may play a part in the development of SM. Although the pattern of behaviour appears distinctive and unique, it can be seen as a heterogeneous phenomenon that may develop in different ways in different circumstances and with different individuals.

TABLE 2.2 FACTORS IN THE DEVELOPMENT
OF SELECTIVE MUTISM

	The community	The family	The child
Disposing factors (Risk Factors)	The family is isolated or marginalized in the community	The parents have personal experience and/or a family tradition of silence/ reticence Factors within the family encourage mutism as a reaction to challenge	The child has the temperamental characteristics of behavioural inhibition Factors within the child favour mutism as a reaction to challenge
Precipitating factors (The trigger)			The child faces a challenging transition to the outside world (or other stressful challenge) and reacts by not speaking in some situations
Maintaining factors (Keeping it going)	Reaction from adults and peers reinforce mutism	Reactions from family members reinforce mutism	The child experiences reduced anxiety and secondary gains

The changing technology of therapy and treatment

In the first report of the successful treatment of SM nearly 80 years ago, Moritz Tramer, a child psychiatrist who worked in the German-speaking area of Switzerland, reported in 1934 on the cure of an eight-year-old selectively mute boy whom he called A. 'During the Easter holidays in 1931 the mother had … received blessed wax from a Capuzin monk to whom she had complained about her son's case. She was supposed to feed the boy from it or sew it into his waistcoat.' On the first day at school after a break the boy said nothing, although he had been told that his parents had accepted the suggestion from the teachers that he should not be allowed to progress to the next grade with his classmates if he did not start talking at school. So they confirmed that he would stay, as agreed, in the second grade. It should also be mentioned that this coincided with a change of teacher.

The mother reported that on that first day she forgot to give A. the blessed wax as intended. 'The next day she made up for it. She said he took the wax 'with delight' On that day he did speak in school, even though only softly. From then on there was progress. After three weeks, during which only one weak relapse occurred, he could be moved up to the third grade where he is now, according to the teacher, the best pupil.' A check-up two years later by a welfare officer indicated that A. was attending fifth grade at grammar school and 'according to his teacher he is a good and hard-working pupil, lively in the lessons, definitely does not exhibit shyness, does not in any way give reason for complaint.' During a home visit the mother reported that 'A. had never had further relapses, was uninhibited with strangers and does all the shopping without any inhibition. She believes that, apart from the wax, the change of teacher at that time and the unpleasant prospect of being moved down had an influence' (Tramer 1934).

Many later observations have supported the view that a change of class or teacher is often associated with a positive shift in patterns of selectively mute behaviour, but that this may not be enough in itself (Cline and Baldwin 2004, pp.99–100). If the blessed wax played a part in A.'s transformation, it will not have been properties of the wax in itself but his understanding of what it represented. In the final section of this chapter I will illustrate changing approaches to the treatment of SM through an examination of the technology associated with them.

The issues and goals that have seemed important to therapists have changed over time. Different theoretical orientations are associated with goals as varied as:

- The child must shape the sounds of speech.

- The boundaries in the child's world must become fuzzier.

- The child must develop the social skills they need for effective communication.

- Others in the family and schools must be helped to allow these developments.

- The child must come to think and feel about speech and silence in different ways.

- The child must develop a new identity – an image of him/herself as a universal speaker.

It might be expected that the use of medication would be targeted simply on reducing general levels of anxiety, but even drug treatments can be conceptualized in different ways according to the practitioner's theoretical explanation of the behaviour. In 1971 it was reported from Ontario, Canada, that a ten-year-old girl called Wilma, who was being treated as an in-patient, was given intravenous injections to help her to 'overcome her presumably strong inhibitions regarding speech'. Although her mute behaviour did not alter, it was noticed that she experienced the injections as a kind of punishment for not speaking – a punishment that she would try to avoid by producing minimal speech. The injection programme was continued with the rule that Wilma could avoid a morning dosage if she met certain speech requirements by bedtime the previous day. The requirements were slowly and systematically increased. 'It appeared that the daily renewed threat situation became a conditioned aversive stimulus, which her speech automatically terminated, resulting in both operant conditioning of her speech and counteraction of the anxiety by aversion relief' (Shaw 1971, p.580).

Thus the medical team in Ontario adapted the drug treatment at their disposal in the service of the behavioural approach to therapy that was current at the time. Later trials of the use of medication in the treatment of SM have tended to focus on the need to reduce overall levels of anxiety, while sometimes exploiting side-effects of some medications that directly facilitate talking (Golwyn and Weinstock 1990). The multi-dimensional causation of SM suggests that medication might be best used as an adjunct to other forms of intervention, but there has been little systematic research comparing the efficacy of either combined approaches to therapy or the outcomes of different forms of medication (Manassis and Tannock 2008; Wong 2010).

Some approaches to treatment evolve not because the process is being conceptualized differently but because improvements in the technology make the original therapeutic goals easier to achieve. This can be seen in the ways that video and audio recording devices can be used to help children who are selectively mute. These were first employed for that purpose over 30 years ago (Dowrick and Hood 1978). The aim was to foster children's perception of their own competence – to help them change their self-image and to develop a new identity as a confident speaker to a wider range of people. The technique is sometimes called self-modelling.

In one example a video recording was made of a child's teacher asking questions in their classroom. The target child made no contribution to the discussion. Then a recording was made using members of the child's family to whom he spoke freely. In that recording family members put to the child the same questions that were put by the teacher in the classroom. This time the child did give oral answers. The two recordings were then edited together to produce a fake video in which the child appears to answer questions competently in the classroom. This was shown several times to the child, who responded by slowly beginning to speak to a wider range of people in school. Following this initial work, others reported the successful use of this type of intervention. Its rationale comes from social learning theory, which would predict that self-modelling will help children to speak because it changes their perception of their own effectiveness.

This approach has a convincing theoretical basis, and the reported success rate is high. It might have been expected that it would be widely adopted and developed further, but in the past the process was a lengthy one, and the technical equipment and expertise were not often easily available to those involved in planning treatment for selectively mute children. Technical changes in consumer electronic equipment mean that that may be changing fast. Whether using audio or video equipment, both the recording and the editing phases are much simpler and quicker than they used to be. Of course, better and cheaper technology is not enough. If video-manipulated self-modelling works, it is not because cameras are smaller and editing is easier; it is because the process draws upon powerful psychological processes. In the end, it is our understanding of SM that has to improve if we are to respond more effectively to the children's needs.

Acknowledgements

This chapter is based on a presentation given to the annual meeting of the Selective Mutism Information & Research Association. I am grateful to Alice Sluckin and the SMIRA Committee for providing the stimulus that led me to reflect back over the last 50 years of work in this field.

CHAPTER 3

Silent Voices

Listening to Some Young People with Selective Mutism and Their Parents

Victoria Roe

The voices of people who have been selectively mute are still largely missing from follow-up reports – and, in fact, from the literature on the subject as a whole.

(Cline and Baldwin 2004, p.213)

This statement became the catalyst for a research project, undertaken as part of an MA course at the University of Leicester (Roe 2011). It aimed to explore the perspectives and experiences of young people and their parents affected by Selective Mutism (SM) and give 'a voice to the voiceless'.

Background

Children with SM are able to speak confidently in some places, but remain silent in others, usually in social situations outside the home. The disturbance lasts longer than one month, excluding the first month at school, and interferes with educational, occupational or social communication. It is not due to a lack of knowledge of, or comfort with, the spoken language required, and is not better accounted for by a communication disorder, pervasive developmental disorder, schizophrenia or other psychotic disorder (APA 1994).

In the past, these children were thought to be stubborn and oppositional, but now it is recognized that many are suffering from an overwhelming anxiety about speaking (Anstendig 1999; Cline and Baldwin 2004; Dow *et al.* 1995). SM was reclassified as an Anxiety Disorder in the *Diagnostic and Statistical Manual-5* (APA 2013).

SM is a relatively rare condition, estimated by Cline and Baldwin (2004) as '6–8 cases of selective mutism per 1000 children through childhood…but…that may well be an underestimate' (p.18). The causes of SM are complex:

> The disorder can result from several diverse pathways reflecting complex interactions between multiple genetic, temperamental, psychological, developmental and social/ environmental systems. The presence of risk and vulnerability factors may predispose certain children to develop SM, but these same factors could also lead to different outcomes.
>
> (Cohan *et al.* 2006, p.351)

Onset often occurs in the early years, when the child begins to move outside the home. Girls are more frequently affected than boys and incidence rates are higher in ethnic minority and bilingual populations. Children with SM may also have various anxiety conditions and there may be a family history of shyness, anxiety, speech and language impairments or psychiatric disorders (Cline and Baldwin 2004; Johnson and Wintgens 2001).

Various methods have been used to treat SM, including psychodynamic, behavioural, therapeutic and family systems approaches. Sometimes different methods have been combined. Since the 1990s there has been some use of drugs in psychopharmacological treatments (Cline and Baldwin 2004).

Research rationale

The UN Convention on the Rights of the Child (United Nations 1989) Articles 12 and 13 asserted the child's right to a voice in decisions affecting them. This principle was incorporated into British law in the Children Act 1989. Since then, there had been a rise of interest in listening to children and young people, including those with vulnerabilities.

However, this change seemed to have had no effect on SM research. Although youngsters and parents provided much of the information for such research, their personal experiences and perspectives were almost absent from the literature, with a few exceptions (Omdal 2007; Omdal and Galloway 2007).

The literature had other deficiencies:

- Few articles contained reports about strategies used by the individual with SM to communicate in situations where they were unable to speak, particularly in school.

- Much of the case study and research evidence on SM was on pre-school or primary school children. Older children were under-represented; even the largest survey in the literature only had 18 subjects aged 12–18 years (Ford *et al.* 1998).

- Sample sizes were generally small, often below 10.

- Studies were usually local; not many covered a wide geographical area.

- Few reports had systematic follow-up of cases.

This study attempted to rectify some of these deficiencies. It used the UK membership of the Selective Mutism Information & Research Association (SMIRA) to conduct an investigation over a wide geographical area, with larger numbers, in the under-researched older age group and provided a means by which the opinions and experiences of children with SM and their parents could be expressed.

Method
Since youngsters with SM have difficulty talking to strangers, an alternative to the interview method had to be found. Omdal and Galloway (2007) had used writing and a computer with three

children in Norway, whilst Ford *et al.* (1998) employed a survey questionnaire in America.

These ideas were combined and two questionnaire surveys, incorporating Likert scales, closed and open questions, were devised and piloted, one for 10–18-year-olds and one for their parents. The questionnaires covered the areas of school, public/social and home/family, as well as SM history and treatment, communication strategies, helps and hindrances, opinions and feelings.

Sample

From the SMIRA membership, 214 potential participants were identified and sent information leaflets and consent forms, of whom 39 requested questionnaires.

This purposive sample may not be representative of all families with SM children, since those who had contacted SMIRA were likely to be the more motivated, articulate and computer-literate parents. However, Ford *et al.* (1998), who drew their large survey sample from the membership of the Selective Mutism Foundation Incorporated in America, explained that this approach 'provided a large sample for a low incidence disorder...that included people from all four regions...from a self-referred, nonclinical organization' which helped reduce 'the referral and severity biases commonly found in samples from particular clinical settings' (p.195). The membership of SMIRA was similarly able to provide a substantial, self-referred sample for this low incidence disorder from across the UK.

The volunteer families returned 30 completed questionnaire sets from England, Scotland and Wales, by post or e-mail, providing a good-sized sample in terms of SM research. The whole 10–18 age range was covered, as was the severity range, from badly affected to fully recovered, making this self-selecting sample sufficiently representative of the SM population for the purposes of this study. Pseudonyms were allocated to protect identities.

The most common family structure was two adults with two children. The majority of parents (84%) and young people (87%)

were white British and spoke English, but 16 per cent of parents and 13 per cent of young people had other ethnicities and were bilingual.

Most young people (83%) attended mainstream school, although two had been home educated in the past, one at Key Stage 2 and one at secondary level. They attended school every day or most days, despite their anxiety about speaking in the school setting. As Adam, aged 10, put it, 'I felt I did not want to go to school because it was scary.' Four respondents were at college and one was not in education, employment or training.

Results

Analysis of the responses confirmed, extended and added new findings to the literature on SM.

Confirmations

This study confirmed many existing SM research findings:

- predominance of females affected: 7M and 23F gave a male–female ratio of 1:3.3

- incidence levels in first-born or only children: 56 per cent

- early onset: for 90 per cent SM began by age 5

- trigger event for SM: 50 per cent, which for 30 per cent was starting nursery/school

- familial shyness patterns: 77 per cent were presently or previously affected

- co-morbid conditions: 60 per cent, of which 40 per cent were anxiety conditions

- incidence levels in bilingual children: 13 per cent of young people

- success of behavioural treatments: 89 per cent in cases using these methods.

(Black and Uhde 1995; Cline and Baldwin 2004; Colligan, Colligan and Dilliard 1997; Crogan and Craven 1982; Dummit *et al.* 1997; Elizur and Perednik 2003; Ford *et al.* 1998; Johnson and Wintgens 2001; Kolvin and Fundudis 1981; Kristensen 2000; Kristensen and Torgersen 2001; Krysanski 2003; Manassis *et al.* 2003; Sluckin *et al.* 1991; Sluckin and Jehu 1969; Steinhausen and Juzi 1996; Vecchio and Kearney 2005.)

Extensions
This study extended existing SM research findings in several areas.

Diagnosis and treatment
Psychologists most frequently diagnosed SM, but teachers, speech and language therapists and parents were also involved in identifying it. Many of those who diagnosed SM were involved in its treatment.

The young people and parents shared their subjective experiences of the professionals involved and the outcomes of the treatments provided. Table 3.1 shows the results.

TABLE 3.1 YOUNG PEOPLE'S AND PARENTS' OPINIONS OF PROFESSIONALS INVOLVED IN SM

	Positive outcome	Negative outcome	Mixed outcome	Totals
Clinical, child and educational psychologists, psychiatrists and psychotherapists	22	10	5	37
Child and Adolescent Mental Health Service	4	7	2	13

GPs, health visitors, family/ local clinics, paediatricians, occupational therapists, school doctors and school nurses	11	6	8	25
Speech and language therapists (SLTs)	15	1	1	17
Teachers and school staff, teaching assistants, SENCOs (Special Educational Needs Co-ordinators) and SEN teachers	33	8	5	46

Examples of good practice in schools included:

- removing the pressure to speak
- allowing parents to support their child in school
- adopting strategies suggested by parents, psychologists and speech and language therapists (SLTs)
- allocating support staff to work with the child
- making special arrangements for break times.

Various treatment strategies were used, successively and in combination. SLTs using behavioural methods were included in the behavioural category. Table 3.2 shows the analysis of responses.

TABLE 3.2 METHODS AND OUTCOMES
OF TREATMENT FOR SM

	Positive outcome	Negative outcome	Mixed outcome	Totals
Behavioural stimulus fading and shaping techniques	17	2	0	19
Speech and language therapy	2	0	2	4
Drugs treatment	3	0	1	4
Cognitive behaviour therapy	1	1	1	3
No pressure to speak	0	0	3	3
Art therapy	2	0	0	2
Home education (at one Key Stage)	2	0	0	2
Psychotherapy	1	1	0	2
One-to-one teaching in school	1	0	1	2
Emotions chart	1	0	0	1
Social skills group in school	1	0	0	1
Play therapy	1	0	0	1
Family therapy	1	0	0	1

Hypnotherapy	1	0	0	1
Homeopathy	1	0	0	1
Healer	1	0	0	1
Behavioural desensitization	0	0	1	1

Behavioural strategies were the most commonly (56%) and successfully (89%) used method. Eight mothers went into school to help their child, usually using behavioural stimulus fading and shaping techniques to enable the child to speak to a widening range of people. Two families had deliberately changed school, to a smaller and more supportive environment, with positive outcomes, facilitating speech.

Communication patterns
The confidence of the young people about speaking in the home, school and public situations was explored by asking them to indicate how often they could talk in those settings.

The presence of close family, friends and relatives made speaking feel easier for the young people both inside and outside the home. For some, speaking was harder when visiting the homes of relatives or friends. In school, more were able to speak to friends than to teachers or support staff. In public, speaking in shops was easier than in any other setting. School, college and places outside the home presented the greatest difficulties, as did strangers, direct questioning or pressure to speak. Three who were able to speak in most places considered themselves to have recovered from SM.

Helps and hindrances
Family and friends were considered most helpful by the young people, who also appreciated their efforts:

Alicia (10 years)
'My Mum invited, one by one, ten girls in the class to play, and then she would ask the girl to sit behind the bed whilst she asked me how to say, for example, dog in Serbian. I felt embarrassed, but after I had done it, pleased.'

Adam (10 years)
'My Mum took me into class after school to talk in Year 2. She showed my story to the teacher. She invited friends home weekly. Having my good friend in the same class helped me a lot.'

Brian (10 years)
'My Mum quit her job to look after me. I have a lot of play dates and met up with a lot of friends after school.'

Eleanor (17 years)
'My Mum and I went out shopping or somewhere every weekend. Gradually I did more and more speaking to people. I did things very slowly that I would never have done before. I feel a lot better and I'm heading in the right direction now.'

Some school staff were also well regarded, as were speech and language therapists and a few psychologists. However, 40 per cent of respondents found school staff to be unhelpful:

Harriet (14 years)
'My tutor. He got me to shout his name as loud as I could and said, "I am not letting you go until you actually shout." I felt humiliated and when I tried to shout, my throat tightened.'

Other respondents also identified pressure to speak and lack of understanding from peers and adults as unhelpful.

Personality and character
The personality characteristics most commonly mentioned in other studies on SM included 'shy', 'withdrawn', 'anxious' and 'stubborn'.

The young people in this study described their personality in their own words. 'Shy', 'quiet', 'introvert', 'unconfident', 'anxious', 'nervous' and 'sad' were mentioned, but by far the majority of descriptors related to positive attributes, such as 'sensitive', 'thoughtful', 'caring', 'kind', 'helpful', 'friendly', 'sociable', 'talkative', 'fun', 'humorous', 'bubbly', 'laughing', 'happy', 'creative', 'artistic', 'studious' and 'sporty'.

Nine of the respondents identified 'introvert' and 'extrovert' qualities in themselves:

Harriet (14 years)
'At home with close family and friends I am: loud, stroppy, happy, sociable and chatty. Outside I am: quiet, anxious and self-conscious.'

The only one to describe herself as 'stubborn' was Eleanor (17 years).

The parents also chose personality descriptors for their children. Again, although 'shy', 'quiet', 'introvert', 'anxious', 'nervous', 'worried' and 'unconfident' were mentioned, they were far outweighed by more positive descriptors such as 'kind', 'thoughtful', 'helpful', 'loving', 'loud', 'sociable', 'confident', 'honest', 'funny', 'sensitive', 'perceptive', 'creative', 'curious', 'hard-working', 'polite', 'wise', 'self-assured', 'happy', 'spirited' and 'talkative'. Parents also identified traits such as 'strength of will', 'determination', 'self-criticism', 'perfectionism', 'a preference for structure/order' and 'control'. Only three parents used 'stubborn'.

Emotional responses such as 'anger', 'frustration', 'aggression', 'moodiness' and even 'depression', displayed by the young people, also featured in the parent's replies:

Mother of Samira (11 years)
'At school, very frustrated and she brings the frustration home. This can change into anger/aggressive behaviour, banging doors, etc., shouting, saying hurtful things.'

The frustration of remaining silent during the school day may account for the emotional outbursts and oppositional behaviour noted in this and some other studies (Ford *et al.* 1998; Steinhausen and Juzi 1996).

The contrasting characters displayed by these young people within and outside the home were also identified by parents.

This evidence of the range of personality characteristics displayed by these particular young people challenges the general perception of those with SM as stubborn, manipulative or merely shy.

New findings

This study added new findings to the SM literature.

Communication strategies

The young people provided evidence of their use of communication strategies, since all but one used non-verbal and 80 per cent used verbal methods. Table 3.3 analyses their responses.

TABLE 3.3 COMMUNICATION STRATEGIES AND RECIPIENTS

	Teacher	Classmate	Relative	Friend	Totals
Gesture/ pointing	20	16	14	10	60
Writing	20	9	4	4	37
Whispering	14	12	6	9	41
Drawing	6	5	3	4	18
Symbol card	8	1	2	1	12
Tape-recording	8	1			9
Message card	4		2		6
E-mail	4	1	3	6	14
Sign language	2	1	1	1	5
Other (speak quietly)	1	1		1	3
Other (talk through friend)	1				1
Social network		6	6	5	17

Computer instant messages		5	3	8	16
Mobile texts	2	6	6	14
Telephone			5	4	9
Webcam				2	2

The most common strategies used were writing, gesture/pointing and whispering. Some strategies were used for specific groups, such as tape-recorder with teachers or telephone with relatives and friends. Mostly, though, a range of different strategies was used with each recipient, demonstrating the determination and ingenuity of the young people in finding methods through which to communicate.

Using techniques such as whispering, audio or video recording and telephoning may be an important stage in the recovery process. However, if the child persists in whispering, then strategies should be employed to increase the volume of speech, in order to avoid possible damage to the vocal cords.

Electronic communication devices were used by 70 per cent and have helped young people with SM to develop their social relationships. For example, two 17-year-olds, Anita, with moderate SM, and Arabella, who had severe SM, used webcams to communicate with their friends.

Paradoxically, technology that distances the speaker from the listener may actually facilitate communication for someone with SM, by reducing the anxiety they experience when face-to-face.

Effects of having SM: school

At school, 80 per cent of the young people thought SM had affected their ability to participate fully in educational and social activities. However, 17 per cent thought SM had not affected them at school and one respondent gave no information.

Martin (11 years)
'I can't be myself.'

Simon (13 years)
'When I know the answer but cannot speak to answer the teacher. I cannot work so well in a group, when I would like to.'

Harriet (14 years)
'I find it hard to socialize and people think I'm a freak because I don't speak much. If I don't understand something, I'm too scared to put my hand up and ask a teacher.'

Arabella (17 years)
'I could not speak in school except for with one close friend. The inability to communicate made me feel vulnerable and fear limited my progress, as I never felt able to express myself in my work. I missed many days when I was too scared to go in.'

Horatia (18 years)
'I couldn't do a lot of subjects, so I had to drop them and I only did three GCSEs. Also I didn't make any friends.'

Two respondents thought SM had not affected them at school, because they had friends, were clever and worked better than others who were always chatting.

The parents confirmed the young people's evidence and revealed that, for 53 per cent, having SM had restricted their learning, progress and options. However, 47 per cent had made good academic progress, despite the limitations of SM, mainly through the support of school staff. In this sample, there was no correlation between severity of SM and academic progress.

Effects of having SM: public/social

Outside school, 70 per cent thought SM had affected them socially, but 27 per cent thought it had not, whilst one respondent gave no information.

Alison (10 years)
'Not talking to certain people; not going to certain places, for example pictures, swimming. I am sick when worried in certain situations.'

Kerry (12 years)
'If I didn't have SM, I'd be more confident and be able to go places and do stuff and have fun.'

Robert (13 years)
'Unable to join in social activity with friends or buy things in shops. Fear of being spoken to when outside the house. Getting lost and unable to ask for directions.'

Emma (17 years)
'I become very anxious when seeing people I know from school outside of school. I am unable to communicate very well with sales people, waiters, etc.'

Horatia (18 years)
'I don't go out much. I just stay home and play on my computer.'

Two respondents thought SM had not affected them socially, because the dancing and sporting activities they enjoyed did not require them to speak.

Again, the parental responses corroborated the young people's experiences. They also revealed that 73 per cent were able to speak to friends in the home, but 27 per cent were unable to do so, being severely affected by SM.

Effects of having SM: home/family

In the family situation, 53 per cent of young people thought SM had affected them, but 40 per cent thought it had not, while two respondents gave no information.

The answers from both parents and young people revealed the impact of a youngster with SM on the household:

Esther (11 years)
'For a long time I wasn't able to speak to uncles and aunts.'

Esther's mother
'A lot of stress on us as parents, especially before we found SMIRA.'

Kerry (12 years)
'I can't talk to certain people in certain situations and it's embarrassing.'

Kerry's mother
'Not always been easy mixing with others as I feel like I have to look out for her all the time to be her voice.'

Anita (17 years)
'I can't talk to some of family, even close. They may feel upset.'

Anita's mother
'Feeling uncomfortable for other people when situations arise and feeling I should apologize for what appears like rudeness.'

Sarah (17 years)
'I don't talk to most family members, so it stops me having a closer relationship with them.'

Sarah's mother
'It has been very hard to understand and help her in the early years. As she got older she could tell us how it was affecting her. Getting information and help from others and online has been very useful to us to try and support, help and understand how to deal with SM and how Sarah deals with each day. We are seeing signs with Sarah in her confidence and try not to push her.'

Other parents also identified 'stress', 'worry', 'frustration', 'lack of understanding' and 'judgement from others' as issues for them.

Mother of Alicia (10 years)
'Lots of stress, worry, constant involvement with school Special Educational Needs Co-ordinator and Speech and Language Therapist (SENCO and SLT). I felt under constant pressure to help her, to do something. My personality changed for a period of time. It required enormous amount of patience. Hardly anyone can understand SM; most people think she can talk but decided not to. It is heart-breaking seeing your child in certain situations when she can't speak.'

Mother of Moira (12 years)
'In the early days we were naturally upset and concerned, a bit frustrated...many times we felt our family didn't support us as grandparents just couldn't get their heads around the situation.'

Mother of Petra (13 years)
'We are worried that she is missing out on friendships and future work prospects. Our son is often asked why his sister doesn't speak, which is difficult for him to answer.'

Mother of Isabelle (13 years)
'We both feel a lot of judgement from others. Comments made by these people can be very hurtful and I think as an SM parent one's own self-esteem can take quite a battering.'

Feelings

Of the young people, 83 per cent provided evidence for the emotional impact of SM on them. Five respondents gave no information. Table 3.4 details their responses.

TABLE 3.4 HOW DOES HAVING SM MAKE YOU FEEL?

	Number
Frustrated, annoyed, angry	8
Different, abnormal, stupid	8
Left out, missing out on life	7
Sad	6
Lonely	5
Wanting to be like others, talk to others	4
Disliked, friendless	4
Embarrassed, uncomfortable	4
Anxious, worried	3
Shy	2
Upset, depressed	2
Physical symptoms of panic	1

cont.

	Number
Wanting to avoid school as it is scary	1
Wanting to hide behind Mum	1
Fine	2

Negative emotions dominated their answers, but the desire to talk was also evidenced. Of the two who felt 'Fine', one had recovered, but one was still severely affected by SM.

Messages and advice

Asked what they would tell others about SM, 80 per cent gave responses, which fell into three categories. Their strongest messages to those without SM were:

> 'I do want to talk, but can't and don't know why. It's not a conscious choice.'

> 'I'm not being rude, arrogant or awkward.'

> 'I'm normal, not dumb or weird.'

> 'It's a disorder, it's different, it's hard.'

> 'It's not just a phase you grow out of.'

> 'I would change if I could, but it's difficult.'

> 'It's hard to speak or join in, due to lack of confidence.'

> 'SM makes people frustrated and angry.'

Their advice to others about helping them was:

> 'Don't make us try to talk or do things; it makes us more anxious.'

> 'Others need to ask if you want to join in activities.'

> 'Don't judge too quickly.'

> 'Be patient and understanding.'

> 'Keep talking to us.'

'Encourage and support us.'

'Make us feel normal.'

'Make no fuss when we don't answer.'

'We'll come round when we feel comfortable.'

Their messages to those with SM were:

'Don't worry or be nervous.'

'You are not alone. There are people who understand.'

'SM may be awful, but you can beat it and have a better life.'

'There is always a way to communicate.'

'Don't be afraid to try and talk. It gets easier the more you do it.'

'Try to whisper or murmur quietly to friends at first.'

'Use SMIRA and *The Selective Mutism Resource Manual*.'

Implications

Their messages have implications for all who have to deal with them.

All professionals need to be better educated about SM and its treatment, as being faced with a silent child can feel threatening and frustrating.

The new evidence from these young people about

- the profound educational, social and emotional impact of SM on them

- their desire to speak but fear of doing so, and

- the way they assess their own characters

may increase our understanding of their motivation and personalities. Their messages about factors and approaches that helped or hindered recovery, and their willingness to use alternative communication strategies, should also inform approaches to treating them.

Early identification and treatment can result in good outcomes, preventing the suffering described by the youngsters and their families in this study (Elizalde-Utnick 2007; Johnson and Jones 2011; Roe 1993). Co-operation between parents and professionals is important for the successful outcome of any treatment programme.

Limitations and future research

This study examined the perspectives and experiences of some young people with SM and their parents from across the UK. Although relatively small and self-selecting, the sample size of 30 was a good number in the context of this rare condition and other SM research studies. Since more than half the sample were aged 10–12, the findings could also be applicable to younger children with SM. These findings would be enhanced by further research into the perspectives of those with SM over a longer period of time and at a younger age. All the families in this study have agreed to follow-up in the future.

Finally

The success of this project in attempting to give 'a voice to the voiceless' was confirmed by Hazel (15 years) in an e-mail when returning her questionnaire:

> 'Thanks for giving me the chance to share my side of the story.'

CHAPTER 4

Setting up a Support Network

Selective Mutism Information & Research Association (SMIRA) – A Brief History

Alice Sluckin, Lindsay Whittington and Rae Smith

In Britain there is a long tradition of charities supporting parents of children with a rare problem. Selective Mutism (SM), previously known as Elective Mutism, is such a problem. Parents have had, and are still having, considerable difficulty finding knowledgeable professionals to support and treat their children, whose problem is that they speak fluently at home but remain silent with strangers in an unfamiliar environment. Though not speaking to their teachers and often not to peers, they are rarely troublesome at school and can easily be overlooked in a busy classroom, despite ongoing parental concern.

In this chapter we would like to describe why and how parents succeeded in setting up a charity to help their children, whose problems, often due to public ignorance, tended to be sadly ignored.

The story starts in Leicester, UK. Alice Sluckin was then a Senior Psychiatric Social Worker at the local Child and Family Guidance Service. In the course of her work she became interested in treating children suffering from SM, successfully using a behaviour modification approach (Sluckin and Jehu 1969; Sluckin 1977). After retiring in 1985 she also worked on a retrospective study of 25 SM children she had treated. Her findings were that those given behavioural programmes with parental support were more likely, on follow-up, to have improved, compared with those given standard school-based remedial programmes from visiting psychologists (Sluckin *et al.* 1991).

As Alice's interest in SM children was becoming known locally, teachers and parents continued to consult her and refer cases to her after she had retired. This is how she came to be approached by Lindsay Whittington, who had been unable to obtain professional help for her selectively mute daughter, despite her best efforts. In 1992 Alice and Lindsay joined forces and started a local support group for parents of SM children and interested professionals. For the parents this was a great relief as they no longer felt isolated, misunderstood and on occasions blamed by teachers.

Parents from as far as Nottingham and Rutland joined the group, which met once a month in a Leicester city school. As time passed the parents became better informed about the condition and appeared less anxious – one of the great contributions of SMIRA. This undoubtedly had a beneficial effect on their children who, it became clear, needed encouragement and to be given time.

A charity is launched

The members of the Leicester Selective Mutism Support group, both parents and professionals, supported by Dr Nigel Foreman and Professor Martin Herbert of the University of Leicester Department of Psychology, were inspired by Lindsay Whittington's enthusiasm for action, and began to think of how they could help all SM children more effectively. Setting up a registered charity came to mind. This, they hoped, would increase public awareness of the condition and also enable them to apply for funding in order to undertake specific projects in the future. With the help of a sympathetic solicitor, the Charity Commission was approached and a draft constitution was submitted. The name of the new charity was to be the Selective Mutism Information & Research Association (SMIRA for short) and the stated objectives in the proposed constitution were as follows:

1. To relieve sickness by providing information on Selective/ Elective Mutism.

2. To support the children's parents and caring professionals.

3. To advance education of the public by conducting research into the condition and making public the results.

On acceptance of the constitution by the Charity Commission, the Selective Mutism Information & Research Association became a registered charity on 30 March 1993. Alice Sluckin was voted Chair and Lindsay Whittington Secretary. Lindsay's past experience as mother of an SM child who had been denied treatment was thought invaluable. She was also a person who showed initiative, perseverance and a great deal of enthusiasm for the cause, as well as having past secretarial experience.

In 1998, after affiliation with 'Contact a Family', it was realized that there was countrywide demand for information about SM, and the Secretary published SMIRA's first newsletter which is now published twice a year and distributed to members. It contains news and reports from parents, as well as book reviews and answers to parents' questions which relate to ongoing difficulties. As it was clear that countrywide ignorance about SM was a major problem, the committee decided to produce handouts giving information about the condition. The first, for professionals, was entitled 'Selective Mutism in Children' (1999, 2008) and the second, for parents, was entitled 'Your Selectively Mute Child' (2000). These were prepared by a chosen working party and contained factual information on SM and suggestions for strategies to be used in the home and at school. They were most competently edited by Victoria Roe, who was a teacher and at one time Special Educational Needs Co-ordinator (SENCO) and is now Deputy Chair of SMIRA.

The handouts continue to be available on request – free of charge and online – and are still very much in demand. They have also been translated into Japanese and French.

In 2002 Alice Sluckin, working jointly with Dr Rosemary Sage (then Senior Lecturer in Special Education at the University of Leicester School of Education), obtained a substantial grant from the (then) Department for Education and Skills to produce a 23-minute video/DVD entitled *Silent Children: Approaches to Selective Mutism*, accompanied by an 84-page informative booklet of the same name (Sage and Sluckin 2004); both were produced by the University of Leicester.

The video and DVD were completed with the help of parents and the University's audio-visual department by 2004. Both the booklet and the video have had excellent reviews and were well received by professionals. For instance, the Social, Emotional and Behavioural Difficulties Association (SEBDA) were happy to promote the materials (Sluckin 2006a). They can be purchased from SMIRA and continue to be in great demand nationally and internationally. Like the handouts, they have been translated into Japanese and French.

In 2007, on receiving a grant from the Yapp Trust, which provides running costs for small charities, the committee was in a position to promote Lindsay Whittington to a part-time paid post as SMIRA Co-ordinator. By then SMIRA had 307 registered parent members and 35 registered professional members. Our charity also offered, at that time, a telephone helpline two evenings a week.

In 2000, as SMIRA was becoming nationally known, the secretary suggested setting up day-long National Parents' Meetings in Leicester and by 2008 these had become established as regular events and are always oversubscribed. Members come from all parts of the country, bringing their children. We have also had parent visitors from abroad. While the parents are busily talking and listening to speakers, the accompanying SM children are encouraged to join supervised children's playgroups. Parents have told us repeatedly that affected children particularly enjoy coming, as they find meeting other SM children therapeutic. In one boy's own words: 'It makes me feel no longer alone.'

This short extract from a report by Julie Brindley, one of our regular childcare helpers, herself formerly SM, will give an indication of the joy of these times:

> After lunch we invited the young people to join in our music-making and singing session. We had a few percussion instruments that enabled us to be creative, noisy and I think

harmonious. Two of the helpers provided us with piano music to play along to. They did a great job, as they had no sheet music but were able to play our requests as well as provide their own ideas.

I remember all too vividly how difficult it could be to go to a strange place...it helps me to empathize with all the young people who came and joined us on Saturday. It took a lot of determination, guts and selflessness to travel, enter the building and be alongside people in such a unique situation, so that parents and carers could attend the meeting.

Other SMIRA activities

There is no charge for membership but parents send voluntary contributions. One of our most successful enterprises was undertaken by members in 2008: this was an Awareness Campaign, suggested by Welsh members and very much supported by Lindsay Whittington. It was undertaken because Welsh members felt that many teachers were still unaware of how to deal with SM children. The campaign was also supported by the Welsh media and the Minister for Education and included production of a special leaflet, 'Not everyone has the confidence to speak everywhere...'. This was written by parents and included an eight-year-old's moving poem as well as a supporter's attractive, colour illustration.

As part of her role as Chair, Alice has written informative papers for professional publications (Sluckin 2000, 2006a, 2006b, 2011). She has also collaborated with our Co-ordinator (Sluckin and Whittington 2009). We have been told that these have been influential and the work is being taken forward with our Deputy Chair (Roe and Sluckin 2014). It is significant that an early paper of Victoria's (Roe 1993) has been widely appreciated, used and quoted.

In 2007 John Bercow MP, now Speaker of the House of Commons, was asked by the UK Parliament to review existing services to children and young people (aged 0–19) with speech, language and communication needs (SLCN). Alice Sluckin, representing SMIRA, was asked to be one of the ten members of the review's chosen

Advisory Group. John Bercow also visited Leicester and met parents of SM children. The Bercow Report (2008) revealed that services for children with SLCN are currently a 'post-code lottery' which cannot be allowed to continue. Hartshorn (2006) pointed out that children's poor communication later carries a high, preventable cost to the nation, and our members can testify to this in terms of social exclusion, mental health and employment difficulties (see, for instance, APA 2013, p.196; Hilari and Botting 2011; Markham and Dean 2006).

A welcome event in 2010 that provided valuable publicity and renewed contacts for SMIRA was the award of an OBE to Alice Sluckin in recognition of her work for the charity.

SMIRA is a member of the Communication Trust, which is a coalition of about 50 voluntary and expert community sector organizations. The Trust launched the National Year of Communication in 2011 with former educational psychologist Jean Gross, CBE, as National Communication Champion for Children. This has encouraged activities designed to ensure that children's communication development remains a national priority. Our Deputy Chair Victoria Roe attends their meetings. SMIRA is thereby involved in such matters as preparation of new legislation and codes of special educational practice.

In 2012 SMIRA participated in a local Afasic (Association for all Speech Impaired Children) 'Voice for Life' conference and Victoria gave a talk derived from her questionnaire-based research among SMIRA families (see Chapter 3) that was very well attended. When Victoria has delivered this talk at further Afasic conferences it has always been well attended, suggesting that the incidence of SM may not be as low as was once thought.

Internet presence

Our Co-ordinator, Lindsay Whittington, describes the road to the development of SMIRA's website:

One particular aspect of parents' meetings had been the sense of enjoyment parents felt at being in contact with others in the same position as themselves. SMIRA was asked if an arrangement could be put in place for them to have contact on a regular basis, possibly by e-mail. Therefore in 2004 a Yahoo! Group smiratalk, now defunct, was set up, allowing parents to communicate by e-mail within the group and access photographs and documents online for the first time. This group became a great success, offering mutual support for parents and direct access to SMIRA's Co-ordinator.

In 2008, with assistance from parent members, SMIRA was able to take advantage of rapidly growing use of the internet and set up its own website. This allowed registered members to gain online access to the handouts and relevant publications and provided a forum, which replaced the earlier 'smiratalk', as a contact point for parents and other interested parties. This website operates today at www.smira.org.uk and welcomes visitors from all over the world, promoting international interest in SM. We are mindful, however, that not everyone has, or even wishes to have, access to the internet. This means that there are still some families who are potentially isolated, or who rely mainly on telephone contact.

Facebook group

With the increased general interest in social media, during 2011 SMIRA took the step of setting up a new group on Facebook. The group gained in popularity during 2012 and at the time of writing has around 1000 members, comprising parents, health and education professionals, teenagers and former sufferers from SM. Members are able to engage in online chat and support each other through shared knowledge and experience, watched over by SMIRA's group administrators.

In 2013 a parent, who is also a primary school teacher with several selectively mute children in her school, posted:

I've commented several times about how much I love this group. I spent almost ten years dealing with my daughter's SM without any support at all. It's so nice to share our journey, all we've learned, and ask for support for the newer things we are encountering. It truly is a lifeline, and one I needed a long, long time ago. Thanks all!

Further developments

We have been glad to support several training days provided by Maggie Johnson on the basis of Johnson and Wintgens (2001). We have also been able to involve local professionals in training days of our own. SMIRA and some of its member families have been involved in several TV documentaries, radio programmes and newspaper articles about SM, which have helped to raise public awareness of the condition and its treatment.

Contributions have been made, in association with Maggie Johnson as a leading expert, to the ongoing revision of its recommendations by the UK National Institute for Health and Care Excellence (NICE) and the US *Diagnostic and Statistical Manual* (*DSM-5*). SMIRA is also contributing to the ongoing revision of the World Health Organization's International Classification of Disorders (*ICD 10*) (WHO 1994).

A Scottish SM group has been established and is linked to SMIRA. Links have been established to other European support groups set up in response to local need using the SMIRA model. We also have connections to Knet, the Japanese internet SM Support Network.

SMIRA would like to acknowledge grants received over the years from:

- Her Majesty's Government (then) Department for Education and Skills

- Rutland Community Foundation

- The Yapp Trust

- Voluntary Action Leicester
- Leicestershire County Council
- Leicester City Council
- Leicester Community Fund.

In 2013 it transpired that Beauty Queen Kirsty Heslewood, who had recently been voted 'Miss England', had at one time suffered from SM and had recovered by means of taking into school an old videotape on which she could be heard speaking. Letting others hear her voice in school seemed to have established her as a potentially communicative person. Kirsty, now completely free of SM, has volunteered to raise funds for SMIRA and was present in Leicester when the charity recently celebrated its 21st birthday.

Finally, we are extremely happy to have Dr Tony Cline, Professor Martin Herbert and Margaret Harrison, CBE (originator of Home Start) as our Patrons and the revered public figure Biddy Baxter, MBE (former editor of the famous BBC children's TV programme *Blue Peter*) as our first President.

Related and Co-morbid
Conditions

CHAPTER 5

Selective Mutism and Communication Disorders

Exploring Co-morbidity

Hilary Cleator

The essence of Selective Mutism (SM) is the absence of speaking in certain situations. Communication disorders such as speech, language and fluency problems may accompany SM. The communication disorder may also contribute to the development of the selectively mute behaviour. An example would be Peter in Chapter 10, whose cleft palate speech may have influenced his willingness to talk in public. The presence of more than one disorder in the same person is called co-morbidity, although the term multi-morbidity has been used recently (Smith 2009). This chapter will explore the existence of communication disorders in children with SM.

Prevalence of communication disorders

It is not entirely clear how many children with SM have a communication disorder. Some studies (e.g. Black and Uhde 1995) have found this occurred in 10 per cent of cases; others (e.g. Krohn *et al.* 1992; Kumpulainen *et al.* 1998) have reported between 30 per cent and 40 per cent of children affected; while more studies (Dow *et al.* 1995; Kolvin and Fundudis 1981; Kristensen 2000) have shown that around half of all children with SM will have some type of communication disorder. The discrepancy between 10 per cent and 50 per cent may occur for several reasons, including small sample size, the population the sample was drawn from (i.e. clinical or community), the study's inclusion criteria, and how the diagnosis was made (e.g. case notes, parental reports, and/or standardized assessments). Furthermore, correctly identifying a communication disorder in children who are usually silent is challenging, although some suggestions will be explored later in this chapter. Currently, there is no consensus about how to test these children's speech and language skills, although it is interesting that studies (e.g. Dow *et al.* 1995; Kolvin and Fundudis 1981; Kristensen 2000) that involved standardized assessments have identified more cases. A recognized formal and comprehensive approach to assessing the communication skills of this population of children is long overdue.

Types of communication disorders

Research into the communication disorders that accompany SM is a work in progress. Early studies have tended to focus on numbers of children affected while some recent papers have provided more detail.

Speech and language

General descriptions are usually given, such as: speech/articulation difficulties, that is, pronunciation problems (Kolvin and Fundudis 1981; Krohn *et al.* 1992) and, language problems (Black and Uhde 1995; Kumpulainen *et al.* 1998; Wong 2010); and speech and language disorder, that is, difficulty using and/or understanding words and grammar (Steinhausen and Juzi 1996; Wong 2010). Not surprisingly, when standardized assessments are administered, more specific information is recorded, such as: phonological delay (Kristensen 2000), which is an immature sound system in word production, for example, 'tar' for 'car', 'pider' for 'spider'; expressive and/or receptive language delay/disorder (Dow *et al.* 1995; Kristensen 2000); and problems with expressive narrative discourse

(Klein *et al.* 2012; McInnes *et al.* 2004). Cases of stammering are also mentioned (e.g. Schwartz *et al.* 2006; Wright *et al.* 1985). For a discussion on stammering, see also Chapter 7. Few research studies have focused just on the communication skills of children with SM when they are speaking – for instance, at home. One exception is an Australian study conducted by the author (Cleator 1998) involving five subjects. Four of the five subjects (three boys and one girl) were found to have a communication disorder, which included: articulation errors; phonological delay/disorder; receptive language disorders; and expressive language problems involving syntax (grammar) and semantics (word meaning). There is still much research needed into this area but, for now, while any communication disorder may be present there is a tendency for problems involving pronunciation and expressive language to be more common.

Children who have a history of speech and/or language problems can also be at risk for difficulties acquiring literacy skills (Harrison *et al.* 2009; Serry, Rose and Liamputtong. 2008). Some studies (e.g. Manassis *et al.* 2007; McInnes and Manassis 2005) have begun to examine this issue as part of their research. To date, there has been a focus on phonemic awareness (the ability to hear, identify and manipulate the sounds in words), which is an important predictor of literacy success. For example, Manassis and colleagues (2007) assessed phonemic awareness as part of a Canadian study that looked at language, cognition and anxiety. They found that the children with SM did not perform as well in this area (and all other language measures) when compared with children in the comparison groups (i.e. those with anxiety but without SM, and a control group). Recognizing that a child with SM may be experiencing additional difficulties with reading, writing and spelling is important because these skills, which can be a source of anxiety at school, are often used during treatment. Currently, literacy remains a largely unexplored area of research in SM.

Voice

Throughout the literature on SM there are references to these children's vocal quality, although actual voice disorders seem not to be reported. Descriptions vary, usually reflecting the setting where the child is speaking. While some parents say their child's voice is loud at home, away from home it's a different matter. Some researchers (Cleator 1998; McInnes and Manassis 2005) report problems with prosody such as volume, intonation and pitch; while others (Kolvin and Fundudis 1981) mention children who say they are afraid of hearing the sound of their voice, or their voice sounds funny (Black and Uhde 1992). Precisely what gives rise to these impressions is difficult to say, but they are not uncommon, so much so that Hayden (1980), in a classification of four types of SM, created a category which she named 'speech phobic mutism' specifically for children who were frightened of hearing their voice. There is no doubt that anxiety may impact on vocal quality (Kagan *et al.* 1987), although the role anxiety plays in the voice of children with SM remains unexplored. Notably, the recent edition of the *Diagnostic and Statistical Manual of Mental Disorders* (APA 2013), hereafter *DSM-5*, has classified SM as an anxiety disorder.

Pragmatics

Of all the communication disorders found in SM, problems with the use of language in social contexts, sometimes referred to as pragmatics, requires the most attention because it is this ability that affects children's inclusion in, or exclusion from, social and academic life. Although it is often difficult to unravel communication behaviours that are attributable to an actual pragmatic disorder from those associated with selectively mute behaviour, these children's communication patterns will reveal both verbal and non-verbal pragmatic problems. For example, opportunities to practise skills such as greeting people, saying 'thank you' and 'sorry', and answering questions, may be absent and possibly undeveloped in a child who is usually silent outside the home.

Non-verbal pragmatic skills may be affected as well, although there seems to be wide individual variation among reported cases. For instance, while some children use gesture to communicate, others avoid eye gaze and have limited facial expression (Lebrun 1990) or appear frozen with fear (McInnes and Manassis 2005) and so anxious they seem physically unable to interact at all (Kanehara *et al.* 2009).

Having said that, there may be a marked discrepancy between social interactions at home and at school, which is important diagnostically for ruling out or clarifying the presence of a pragmatic disorder. For example, while some children will be inhibited at school, at home they may display impulsive and/or oppositional verbal behaviour (Cunningham *et al.* 2004) with some parents reporting that they are overly talkative (Lebrun 1990). By contrast, other children may continue to be reticent at home, often reflecting their family's culture of quietness (APA 2013; Steinhausen *et al.* 2006). This is one of the problems in researching SM because there is considerable individual variation (Cline and Baldwin 2004). Studies often do not include large numbers of cases because the condition is rare, which results in conflicting findings that make it difficult to generalize to a wider population.

Speech and language development and onset of selectively mute behaviour

Most parents of children with SM report no problems with their child's early speech and language development (i.e. during the first year). It is when the child starts using language to communicate during the second year that delay is sometimes mentioned (Kolvin and Fundudis 1981; Toppelberg *et al.* 2005). For example, Kolvin and Fundudis (1981) reported that the 24 children with SM in their English study began using phrases five and a half months later (27.3 months compared with 21.9 months) than the 102 matched control group; and Cleator (1998) found that four of the five subjects in her study had a history of delayed speech and language development.

Of further interest in the (admittedly small) study conducted by the author was the parents' observation that, for no apparent reason, the speech and language development in three of the four subjects appeared to stop between the ages of 12 and 18 months and, although it had resumed, had never become normal.

Parents usually state that the selectively mute behaviour started in the pre-school years, which coincide with a period of rapid growth in a child's speech and language development. It is at this time that communication skills are at their most vulnerable and problems such as stammering are most likely to develop. It is possible that some form of disruption or stress during this period may impinge on the child's developing communication skills. For instance, separating from a caregiver is a challenging experience for most children who are often shy and withdrawn when they start daycare or pre-school, with some experiencing separation anxiety (Black and Uhde 1995; Steinhausen and Juzi 1996) after being left on their own, often for the first time. For most children, these feelings pass. However, for some, remaining silent may help them reduce feelings of anxiety and perhaps signal the beginning of the selectively mute behaviour.

With transition to school, the child's coping skills will once again be challenged. Whereas at home a child can speak spontaneously, it is the teacher who controls most of the talking in the classroom. To compound the problem, differences exist between language spoken at home and at school. For example, children have to learn how to answer the teacher's questions, and stand up in front of the class and give news. They also have to learn to master narrative discourse such as telling stories, sharing experiences and giving explanations (Sage 2004). Not only will being silent reduce opportunities to learn and practise these linguistic skills (Klein *et al.* 2012; McInnes and Manassis 2005) but there will be social implications, too. For instance, the child will miss out on chances to develop relationships through activities involving language such as negotiating with peers, discussing events or programmes on TV, and telling jokes. Some children may even be teased (Cline and Baldwin 2004; APA 2013) or picked on by other children because they are unable to protect themselves verbally (Manassis 2009). It is not difficult to see how a child with SM and a communication disorder will be doubly disadvantaged.

A communication disorder as an area of vulnerability

Why might children develop a fear of speaking? One answer is that, for some, talking is an area of vulnerability because of a communication disorder. This view is not new. As early as 1912, Gutzman (1912, cited in Kratochwill 1981) proposed that SM may develop as a reaction to being teased, criticized or not understood because of a speech and/or language problem. More recently, others (e.g. Elizur and Perednik 2003; Klein *et al.* 2012) have supported the idea that a communication disorder could be a factor in the development of the selectively mute behaviour. Certainly, children who have difficulties expressing themselves verbally and whose speech is sometimes unintelligible are likely to feel worried about speaking, especially at school. Such children may remain silent in an attempt to reduce feelings of anxiety (Anstendig 1998). Indeed, the development of anxiety along with social isolation, withdrawal and reticence has been found among children with language problems (McInnes and Manassis 2005), especially those with expressive language delay (Irwin, Carter and Briggs-Gowen 2002).

Meanwhile, other researchers (Elizur and Perednik 2003; Kristensen 2000) have gone further and suggested that the communication disorder could be part of an underlying neurodevelopmental immaturity that makes the selectively mute child vulnerable to everyday challenges. For example, Kristensen (2000), in a Norwegian study of 54 children with SM, found that 68.5 per cent met the criteria for a diagnosis of developmental delay/disorder (motor, language) compared with 13 per cent of the 108 children in the control group. The observation that multiple factors may be implicated in the development of the selectively mute behaviour led Steinhausen and Juzi (1996) to propose a vulnerability model for the development of the disorder. There will be important treatment implications if this is the case, because the silent behaviour may be concealing other co-morbid conditions such as a disabling communication disorder (Kristensen 2000). By attempting to treat just the selectively mute behaviour, clinicians will be missing other problems which require attention if a full recovery is to be possible (Elizur and Perednik 2003). In this connection, it is worth mentioning the issue of gender. SM seems to occur more often among girls (Kumpulainen *et al.* 1998; Steinhausen and Juzi 1996) whereas communication disorders are more commonly found among boys (McLeod and McKinnon 2007). It therefore seems likely that more boys than girls with SM will have a communication disorder and clinicians should be mindful of this. The need for future studies to identify the sex of subjects with co-morbid problems is recommended.

Before proceeding further, it is relevant to look at two groups where there is an increased incidence of SM: children from migrant families and twins.

SM and children from migrant families

Studies (Elizur and Perednik 2003; Toppelberg *et al.* 2005) have clearly demonstrated that children from migrant families are more at risk for developing SM than children from non-migrant backgrounds. Some children either do not learn the native language prior to school entry or have difficulty mastering the new language, especially if they have a communication disorder. In many ways, early second language acquisition resembles a communication disorder with the likelihood of mispronunciations, grammatical errors and prosodic deviation (e.g. speaking with an accent). It is easy to see how concerns about being teased for the way they speak might make a child feel shy and self-conscious about talking, especially in front of peers (McInnes and Manassis 2005). Some children may even stop speaking for a while (Toppelberg *et al.* 2005), although the duration and even existence of what has sometimes been referred to as 'the silent period' has been questioned by some (Gibbons 1985). The migration process is complex so it would be misleading to suggest that the increased incidence of SM among children from migrant backgrounds is due solely to issues involving second language acquisition. Nevertheless, it is entirely understandable how learning a second language, together with starting school, could be challenging experiences for some children.

SM and twins

While twins represent around 1.1 per cent of all live births, the occurrence of SM among twins in the general population is difficult to calculate. Cline and Baldwin (2004), using the numbers of twins featured in the published (English) literature on SM, estimated a minimum incidence of around 4 per cent. Twins with SM usually speak to each other, but sometimes not at home with family members (Wallace 1986). Obviously, twins have a different language experience from singletons. For example, two-way communication is regularly extended to include a third party, thereby reducing occasions for one-on-one conversational exchanges; and twins spend a lot of time speaking to one another, possibly limiting the scope of their language experience.

While twins' language acquisition usually follows a similar pattern to that of singletons, delay between the ages of two and four has been reported, although this has usually resolved by the time the twins reach the ages of seven and eight (Crystal 1997). In cases where there is a communication delay or disorder, twins may inadvertently reinforce each other's non-standard speech and language behaviour, with some continuing to use these features beyond an age when they are appropriate. Indeed, the development of so-called secret languages may, in fact, emerge from these communication patterns (Crystal 1997). It is possible that some of the different language behaviours observed among twins may become a means for maintaining the self-sufficiency of the twinship and contribute to the formation of SM in some cases.

Pathways and a biopsychosocial model

So far, this chapter has focused on SM and communication disorders. It would be misleading to imply the presence of just one co-morbid condition, because any number may be present (Kristensen 2000; Manassis *et al.* 2007). For example, in a Japanese study conducted by paediatrician Kanehara *et al.* (2009), the following co-morbid conditions in 23 cases of SM were found: anxiety disorders (73.9%); developmental disorder (60%); other disorders such as bedwetting. (The study was published prior to the classification of SM as an anxiety disorder in *DSM-5*.) This was a clinical sample and the 'symptom burden', as Kristensen (2000) has called it, among cases in the wider community may not be as heavy. There is no doubt that some cases of SM have a greater number of co-morbid conditions than others, and with this comes complexity. In such cases the term multi-morbidity seems more appropriate (Smith 2009).

The complexity often found in cases of SM has led some researchers to try to harness the elusive nature of the disorder by creating sub-groups. Some studies (Cohan *et al.* 2008; Kristensen and Torgersen 2001) have included the presence, or not, of a communication disorder. For example, Cohan and colleagues (2008) identified three groups of children: (1) those who were mildly anxious when pressured to speak; (2) those who were just anxious; and (3) those who were anxious and had delayed communication skills. Cohan and associates suggested that this latter group could be 'the most severely impaired' (Cohan *et al.* 2008, p.780). More research is required to explore this issue.

Children with SM are a diverse population, so creating sub-groups has its difficulties. Another approach is to view the behaviour – that is, not talking – as a symptom of a wide range of disturbances, and the diagnosis of SM an umbrella term for grouping together children with differing pathologies (Anstendig 1998; Kumpulainen *et al.* 1998). Indeed, the presence of multi-morbidity in SM has led several writers (Elizur and Perednik 2003; McInnes and Manassis 2005) to suggest that there may be different pathways leading to the development of the silent behaviour. In order to conceptualize these pathways, a broad framework is helpful, especially clinically. One such framework is the biopsychosocial model proposed by Engel (1980) which examines biological, psychological, and social factors (see Figure 5.1, page 92).

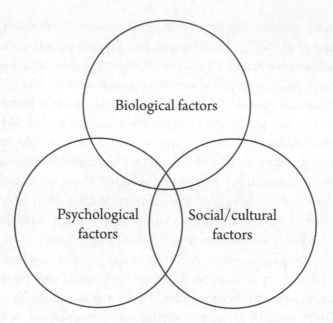

Figure 5.1 The biopsychosocial/cultural model

Recently, the model has been extended to include cultural factors, making its application to SM all the more pertinent because of the often compelling role cultural factors play, especially among children from migrant backgrounds. Applying a biopsychosocial model should clearly demonstrate where the 'symptom burden' (Kristensen 2000, p.254) lies. For example, a child with neurodevelopmental immaturity will have more biological features than a child from a migrant background who will likely have more social/cultural factors. This will assist in preparing each child's unique formulation during assessment.

Assessment and treatment

Children with SM are best managed by a multi-disciplinary team (Dow *et al.* 1995; McInnes *et al.* 2004). This could include a paediatrician, clinicians with a background in mental health such as a psychiatrist and/or clinical psychologist, and a speech and language therapist.

Assessment

Assessment usually involves a full case history from parents so that issues such as the child's developmental milestones, medical history, patterns of socialization and progress at school can be explored. If the history reveals the existence of other conditions such as developmental and/or behavioural problems, referral to an appropriate specialist can be made (Keen, Fonseca and Wintgens 2008). As far as the child's speech and language development is concerned, it is not adequate to rely solely on parental reports, and referral to a speech and language therapist is essential (Dow *et al*. 1995; Wong 2010), especially when the parent interview reveals a family history of communication disorders (Cohan *et al*. 2008; McLaughlin 2011). If the child is from a migrant background, it is necessary to make sure sufficient time has passed to allow familiarity with a new language to develop. If the child has had at least six months' exposure to a new language but is still mute, a bilingual speech and language therapist who speaks both languages, or an experienced interpreter, should be found to conduct the assessment (Toppelberg *et al*. 2005). The child's hearing should also be tested (Cleator 1998; Wong 2010) and an oromuscular assessment carried out, although some children with SM are hesitant about opening their mouths (Cleator 1998; Lebrun 1990), so sensitivity is required.

Conducting a comprehensive speech and language assessment of children who are usually silent is complicated. Nevertheless, an assessment is possible if it is conducted under certain conditions. Administering standardized language comprehension tests is usually straightforward because the child does not have to speak. However, assessing the speech and expressive language of children who are usually silent involves some creativity, especially on issues such as who does the testing and where.

Some successful methods include:

- obtaining from the family audio- and/or videotapes of the child speaking at home for later transcription and analysis (Cleator 1998; McInnes and Manassis 2005)

- training parents to administer tests either at home or in the clinic using a one-way mirror (Cunningham *et al.* 2004; Klein *et al.* 2012; McInnes and Manassis 2005)

- conducting the assessment in the setting where the child usually speaks and feels comfortable, namely their home (Cleator and Hand 2001; Cohan *et al.* 2008).

Whether a child will speak during assessment in a clinical setting is unpredictable. Klein and colleagues (2012) looked at this issue and found that all 33 children in their American study spoke during testing when they were alone with their parents but only 18 spoke when the tests were administered by a speech and language pathologist. The study also found that children scored higher when tests were administered by parents. It is not always possible to obtain an accurate picture of the child's true communication skills during the first contact because their performance may be influenced by anxiety and behavioural inhibition, so further attempts may be necessary. A number of researchers (Dow *et al.* 1995) have suggested tests that could be used with this population of children, while others (e.g. McInnes and Manassis 2005) have provided information for conducting a comprehensive, standardized assessment of these children's speech and language skills. Furthermore, there is no doubt that social media (e.g. Skype, Vine) will make an increasing contribution not only to their assessment but to their treatment, too.

Treatment

Treatment of the selectively mute behaviour will ideally involve a multi-disciplinary team that includes members of the child's family and their teacher. Obviously, the teacher, who is often most affected by the selectively mute behaviour, will play a critical role during treatment. Unfortunately, little research has focused on exploring that role from a teacher's perspective.

Therapy for the communication disorder may begin and continue simultaneously with treatment of the selectively mute behaviour (Klein *et al.* 2012; McInnes and Manassis 2005). Having said that, some clinicians (McInnes and Manassis 2005; Smayling 1959) have found that focusing just on the communication disorder can have positive effects on reducing the selectively mute behaviour itself. This finding is intriguing. It is beyond the scope of this chapter to explore what mechanisms could be involved here but, it is hoped, further clinical experience and research will shed light on the issue.

Even if the child does not have a diagnosable communication disorder, a case may be made for involving a speech and language therapist in developing the child's essential pragmatic skills so they gain confidence speaking socially (McLaughlin 2011). This may include practising routines such as offering an opinion, asking questions, interrupting politely and taking conversational turns in an acceptable way (Dow *et al.* 1995). Even after the elimination of selectively mute behaviour, support and encouragement is likely to be necessary so the children consolidate their gains and continue to develop communication skills as they increase the number of people they speak to and where they speak. Thus, maintenance of a level of communicative competence and generalization of speaking to other settings will require ongoing support for some children.

A final word on intervention

Early intervention is essential in SM (Kanehara *et al.* 2009; Keen *et al.* 2008; Schwartz *et al.* 2006). Unfortunately, there are many instances reported in the literature (Kumpulainen *et al.* 1998; Steinhausen and Juzi 1996) where a substantial time-lag exists between the onset of the selectively mute behaviour and beginning of treatment. For example, Schwartz and colleagues (2006) found a period of 11.5 months between the time when parents voiced their concerns to their doctor and when a diagnosis was made. They also found that 69.7 per cent of the children in their American study had never been diagnosed correctly nor referred for intervention. One of the reasons may be acceptance of shyness and reticence in children at the time the behaviour is usually first noticed (i.e. aged between three and five years).

Clearly, most children overcome being silent but a small number do not. Regrettably, at the moment there appears to be no way of distinguishing between the two groups. It is always important to remember that these are vulnerable children for whom facing life outside the home is challenging. Rather than adopting a 'wait and see' policy, a proactive approach would be to refer any child who shows signs of assuming a silent position for assessment as soon as possible (Schwartz *et al.* 2006). Personnel working in the area of childcare are ideally placed to make this referral, and they are also in a position to refer children with a communication disorder. For, while a communication disorder is neither necessary nor sufficient for the development of SM, in some cases it may be one of a number of co-morbid conditions that lays the foundation for the development of the selectively mute behaviour.

Acknowledgements

I would like to acknowledge the many helpful discussions with Dr Peter Jenkings, Professor Vicki Reed, Professor Mark Onslow and especially Dr Linda Hand. Also, the assistance of Christine Monie, librarian.

CHAPTER 6

Exploring the Relationship of Selective Mutism to Autism Spectrum Disorder

Alison Wintgens

A child is seen standing alone in the playground looking worried and rather sad. S/he is said to be socially isolated, wary of changes or new things, rather a perfectionist and talking very little. School staff are concerned. Could s/he have an autism spectrum disorder, or Selective Mutism (SM), or both, or some other anxiety or communication disorder? In this chapter we will consider common misconceptions and misdiagnoses of SM, the similarities and differences between SM and autism spectrum disorders (ASD), and look at how common it is for these two to co-exist. We will discuss the issues that may arise in diagnosis of the two conditions, and guidelines and pitfalls of assessment. Suggestions will be made for management of SM if a child or young person has the dual diagnosis.

Common misconceptions and misdiagnoses

There is no doubt that people still do not fully understand SM, and they may either confuse it with or miss other diagnoses. Many people have never come across SM in spite of developments in the past ten to fifteen years, increased coverage in the media and in the literature of professionals, and the splendid work done in various countries by voluntary organizations such as SMIRA and the Selective Mutism Foundation in the USA. In some ways it is a hidden difficulty and usually temporary, and it may seem perplexing to some since the mutism does not occur in every setting with all people.

Diagnosis of childhood disorders is a complex and subtle business. Issues and misunderstandings may arise from inadequate experience or knowledge about the field of differential diagnosis, and this can apply to educational and medical professionals and therapists as well as the general public. Some people do not understand exactly what features are necessary for the diagnosis of a certain condition, or that many conditions have overlapping symptoms, or that a child or young person may have more than one diagnosis. Regrettably, when a child may possibly have more than one diagnosis, there can sometimes be a blinkered attitude to assessment, a failure to look broadly and deeply enough at all the symptoms or to see the child or young person as a whole.

So what are the most common misconceptions and misdiagnoses and the ensuing problems that can occur? Up to 20 years ago SM was called Elective Mutism and generally thought of as wilful and deliberate refusal to talk, leading to an assumption – if not a diagnosis – of a behaviour disorder. The child's silence received a lot of attention, pressure was put on the child to talk, unrealistic rewards or bribes were offered and sometimes punishment or penalties might have been exacted if the child did not progress. Of course this can still happen. However, as a result of more accurate and widespread publicity and research, more people now understand that it is an anxiety disorder, and its new classification as such in the *Diagnostic and Statistical Manual,* 5th edition, *DSM-5* (APA 2013) is a great help. However, some people may recognize it as an anxiety condition but continue to misunderstand the cause. Suspecting that the SM is a result of specific trauma or abuse or solely due to an attachment disorder, they may adopt a rather blaming attitude and may unhelpfully refer the child in the first instance for a form of psychotherapy.

Other difficulties may occur with possible speech, language and communication disorders or problems with dual language or ESOL

(English for Speakers of Other Languages). Assumptions can be made that these are the reasons for the lack of talking. The SM is then overlooked, rather than advice sought from a speech and language therapist or an ESOL specialist as to the existence and relationship of SM with one of these problems.

Lastly there are misconceptions and misdiagnoses around SM and ASD. Most commonly questions are asked as to whether children (before or after a diagnosis of SM) who do not communicate or make eye-contact may have ASD; or whether older children whose SM has not resolved as expected may have ASD.

Features of ASD and SM

In considering the issues that arise around the diagnosis of both SM and ASD, and the reasons for possible confusions, it is necessary to be clear about the key features of the two conditions. We start by looking at summaries of the recently published *DSM-5* and note the modifications of the classification of both from the previous edition. Many readers, and of course those carrying out assessment, are advised to look at the exact words that appear in *DSM-5*.

Autism Spectrum Disorder can be recognized by the early onset of features in two areas:

1. Persistent deficits in social communication and social interaction across multiple contexts, incorporating the two areas previously described in *DSM-IV* as social impairment/ reciprocal interaction and communication impairment. These deficits are divided into three sub-groups. First, deficits in social-emotional reciprocity, which covers: abnormal social approach and failure of normal back-and-forth conversation; reduced sharing of interests, emotions or affect; and failure to initiate or respond to social interactions. The second sub-group is deficits in non-verbal communication, covering eye contact, body language, gestures and facial expressions. Third, we have deficits in developing, maintaining and understanding relationships, looking at difficulties adjusting behaviour to suit

various social contexts, sharing imaginative play or making friends, and absence of interest in peers.

2. Restricted, repetitive patterns of behaviour, interests or activities, previously known as restricted and repetitive activities and interests. There are four sub-groups of symptoms in this area. One relates to stereotyped or repetitive motor movements, use of objects or speech; another to insistence on sameness, routines, or ritualized patterns of verbal or non-verbal behaviour; another to abnormally intense and highly restricted, fixated interests; and the fourth to hyper- or hypo-reactivity to or unusual interest in sensory input.

All three social communication and social interaction deficits must be evident, whereas only two of the four restricted, repetitive patterns of behaviour, interests or activities need to be present. An interesting change to note since *DSM-IV* is that the presence of the symptoms is now evaluated by three specific severity levels based on the level of support required, with examples given as to what this means in practice.

ASD is now a single diagnostic category so, following research into the inconsistency of distinctions among the various ASD subtypes, Asperger Syndrome is not included in *DSM-5*, nor are the other two less well known sub-diagnoses Pervasive Developmental Disorder Not Otherwise Specified and Disintegrative Disorder.

Selective Mutism is for the first time classified in *DSM-5* under Anxiety Disorders, which is a clear statement and should be a great help when parents and others are trying to explain about the fundamental nature of the disorder. The wording of the five diagnostic criteria has not changed in the new edition. The main feature remains the consistent failure to speak in specific social situations despite speaking in other situations; and the second notes the effect of this on educational or occupational achievement or with social communication. SM can be diagnosed after a month, provided this is not the first month of school. The last two features state that the lack of knowledge or comfort with the required spoken language, or a disorder of communication such as stammering or a condition such as ASD, are not the cause and do not explain the mutism. Put another way, SM is more than the silences that all children with speech and language impairment, stammering or ASD may exhibit at times, although it is important to remember that these other diagnoses may also be present, as is discussed further in the next section.

Co-existence of ASD with SM

Co-existence (or co-morbidity, which is the medical term) is common in the field of developmental disorders, so it is not surprising that some children and young people with SM have also been found to have additional difficulties and diagnoses. In *The Selective Mutism Resource Manual* (2001), Johnson and Wintgens attempted to break down the diagnostic categories of SM into four sub-groups. Box 6.1 shows the three categories they currently use based on more recent experience. Using this framework, children and young people with an additional diagnosis of ASD would come under the category of 'Complex Selective Mutism'.

BOX 6.1 JOHNSON AND WINTGENS' DIAGNOSTIC CATEGORIES OF SELECZTIVE MUTISM

- *Pure Selective Mutism*, where children have no additional disorders. It may be termed 'low or high profile' depending on whether the presentation is obvious.

- *Selective Mutism, plus speech* or *language impairment* or *ESOL (English as a Second or Other Language)* problems.

- *Complex Selective Mutism* – SM plus other diagnoses such as ASD or SAD (Social Anxiety Disorder), or significant major concerns (medical, environmental or emotional).

One of the most comprehensive studies of co-morbidity that mentions ASD (in the form of Asperger Syndrome) is that of Kristensen (2000), who looked at 54 children and young people with SM matched by 54 controls. She found 69 per cent with one or more additional developmental disorders, whereas this occurred in only 13 per cent of the controls. Of the 69 per cent, 7 per cent were said to have Asperger Syndrome; and 74 per cent had additional anxiety disorders compared with 7 per cent in the control group. Most strikingly, 46 per cent of those in the SM group had both a developmental disorder *and* an anxiety disorder, which only applied to 1 per cent of the control group.

Could it be more than SM?

In the author's experience, questions of possible dual diagnosis mostly arise about whether a child with SM may also have ASD or some other disorder rather than the reverse. This is probably because initial or superficial diagnosis of SM is not difficult and can generally be made early. Essentially, the child or young person will consistently speak freely to some people in some situations (usually to close family members at home) and not to others in less familiar situations. Many who work with and observe this in pre-school or school-age children will recognize it as SM. It may help at this stage to have the diagnosis confirmed by someone with more experience of SM, but it is not essential to have an 'official' diagnosis of SM before putting some strategies in place to help the child.

Clearly, there are some children whose SM does not resolve as expected; they do not make much progress with talking fully and freely to more people or they appear to have reached a plateau. Rather than immediately looking for a possible second diagnosis, it is wise to consider a more in-depth assessment of the SM and to look thoroughly at why the SM interventions may not be working. The advanced training in SM at University College London addresses common practices that prevent or hinder progress, the first of which relates to inadequate assessment of the SM. Quite often it is found that unexplored factors at home or school are reinforcing the child's mutism or raising her anxiety, or that cultural or personal inhibitions may be present. With some children there is not sufficient appropriate intervention, or it is not broken into small enough steps or carried out frequently enough. These issues all need to be addressed in the first instance. Of course, the child may indeed have additional problems such as ASD, an attachment disorder or other anxiety or communication disorder, and it would be prudent at this stage to consider all these options. The school psychologist or speech and language therapist should look at a broader and deeper assessment of the concerns, possibly using the Parental and School Interview Forms from *The Selective Mutism Resource Manual* (Johnson and Wintgens 2001). This may then indicate the need for further referral and which specialist or team might best be able to undertake appropriate assessment and diagnosis.

Possible similar symptoms in SM and ASD

There is no doubt that children and young people with SM appear to present with some similar symptoms to those with ASD, partly because some anxiety-based behaviours can look very much like autism. It may be that this can lead to misunderstandings or misdiagnoses. However, a more detailed look at the symptoms is likely to show that they occur for different reasons or they manifest in somewhat different ways. Let us look at the various features and consider why they may arise and whether they really are similar in the two conditions.

Reluctance to communicate

At first glance in a situation such as school, children with SM and those with ASD both seem reluctant to communicate. On closer inspection we see that children with SM have a specific pattern of non-communication which is person- or situation-related, but have normal reciprocal conversation with people in their comfort zone. In contrast, children with ASD often don't talk much to close family either. They don't do social chit-chat because they don't see the point of it and need to be really interested in something before it stimulates their desire to talk. Their reluctance to communicate is topic-related rather than person-related.

Wariness of change or things that are new or different
Children with either of the two conditions do not cope well with the unexpected. For example, in school something like a change in the timetable or a different teacher may cause them to be upset as they prefer structure and certainty. For those with SM this is triggered by their anxiety: there may be new people who don't understand about SM or they may be expected to speak more than they are able. Sufferers of ASD, however, prefer things to be the same because they are confused by change; new things don't make sense to them and disrupt the safe routine that they need.

Social isolation
If observed in unfamiliar and group situations, someone with SM may appear socially isolated because of the fear of having to talk, but once the child is within her comfort zone she will not appear isolated. An example of this can be seen in the *Silent Children* DVD (2004, available from SMIRA) when Rachel is at home at a birthday party for her grandmother. In contrast, those with ASD will appear isolated or socially different to their peers even with familiar people in familiar settings, because of their social communication deficits.

Problems with social skills
There is no doubt that children with SM lack experience of developing social skills in the usual way. They cannot manage to use everyday greetings and terms of politeness with unfamiliar people. They cannot experience talking and then having to keep quiet at certain times in nursery or practise sharing or working in groups in school. For these reasons it is sometimes necessary, once their SM has resolved, for them to have some training in assertiveness or social skills, or informal help in this area from parents and school. In contrast, a child with ASD, despite social skills training through which he might learn new skills, is always likely to have difficulty in this area. This is part of the condition, the reason he has an ASD diagnosis.

Desire to get things right

Perfectionism is a trait that has been noted in children with either SM or ASD. The child with SM is cautious, restrained and tends not to take risks. This seems to arise out of self-consciousness, because of anxiety about drawing attention to themselves or being criticized. In contrast, the child with ASD is not self-conscious but his actions are governed by rigidity, concrete thinking and inappropriate attention to detail.

Differences in eye contact

The quality and quantity of appropriate eye contact is noticeable in children with either of these two conditions. Because of their anxiety and the wish to avoid talking, children with SM are often seen to be wary and watchful, they may appear to stare in rather a frozen way, or they may look down. In a child with ASD the quality of eye contact is unusual during communication: most often there is a lack of eye contact when speaking or listening, or the eyes are not used for referencing, that is, not directed towards what the child is talking about and back to check that the listener is following.

Differences in body posture

Again, the differences in body posture are displayed in different ways in the two conditions. The child with SM, when out of his/her comfort zone, will appear tense, frozen or stiff, like a rabbit trapped in the headlights. Tension may be manifest in raised shoulders or turning the whole of the upper body rather than just turning the head. Sometimes body posture is so extreme or bizarre that children have been referred to a physiotherapist. Body posture in someone with ASD looks different: it occurs in the form of mannerisms or stereotyped body movements. As with social isolation, children with SM have normal eye contact and body posture once they are in their comfort zone, in contrast to children with ASD.

Difficulty with open questions

A child with SM is anxious about talking with unfamiliar people and has to gradually build up competence and confidence in small steps. It is easier if this is practised in tasks where there is a low communication load – where speech is automatic or rote-learnt, simple and concrete or a short answer to a closed question, as opposed to tasks with a high communication load where the child has to express personal, uncertain or controversial opinions. In contrast, the child with ASD has intrinsic problems with abstract language, and is rigid and concrete in his thinking; these are the reasons why he/she copes better with closed questions or when given limited choices.

Guidelines and pitfalls in the assessment of ASD in a child with SM

An assessment for the right reasons

An assessment of possible ASD is important and helpful for several reasons. If confirmed, it may help people understand the pattern of behaviours the child is presenting; it may explain the additional concerns parents have sometimes had for a long while, and the 'label' may point the family and school towards more appropriate strategies than have been offered so far. Sometimes it may affect the level of support the child receives or even his/her educational placement. The reverse is also true. If a diagnosis of ASD is not confirmed, this can also put an end to the mis-labelling of the child. However some may be disappointed that there is no label, no fresh start and possibly no increased help. Indeed, regrettably, it has been known for people to recommend or seek an ASD diagnosis thinking that they can access more help for the child than they have been offered with 'only a diagnosis of SM'.

General guidelines and comments

Let us assume that a decision has been made, for the right reasons, to consider whether the child or young person may have ASD. The suggestions below apply equally to children being assessed for ASD as a first diagnosis when in fact they may well have SM but this hasn't been identified or a second diagnosis to see whether the child or young person with SM may also have ASD. Where and how this is done will obviously depend on local services, but below we will consider guidelines of what makes for a thorough assessment. Questions need to be asked about the contents of the assessment, the assessors' experience and understanding of SM, and the modifications that will need to be made when assessing ASD in a child with possible or identified SM. This is important since SM is rarely seen in specialist paediatric or mental health clinics. In addition, the ASD may not be very obvious or it would have been picked up earlier.

Involvement of several professionals

It is good practice when assessing a child with a possible ASD for more than one professional to be involved. The professionals need experience and expertise in developmental, behavioural and communication disorders, so most usually it will be a paediatrician or child psychiatrist, plus psychologist and/or speech and language therapist. The assessment may be done by a team in a Children's Centre, Developmental Paediatric or Child and Adolescent Mental Health setting, and they may hold a special clinic for the purpose.

A typical assessment

In order to decide whether a child may have ASD, the assessor needs to get a detailed history of the child's development, behaviour and experiences, as well as a picture of the child's current presentation. This is achieved in two ways: it is based on information from those who know him well, and also from meeting, observing and communicating with the child himself. An interview with the parents or carers may be the sole method of gathering the information, but questionnaires may also be used, and there may be reports from others who know the child well, such as school staff.

Specific assessment measures

The Autism Diagnostic Interview – Revised (ADI-R) (Rutter *et al.* 2003) is a tool that is commonly used to gather information from parents or carers about children over the age of two years. The ADI-R is a standardized semi-structured interview that is scored. When used to assess whether a child who is mute with strangers may have ASD, it has the advantage that the parent or carer can comment on the child's behaviour with familiar people in a familiar, comfortable setting. Allowances should be made for the limited social experiences of the child with SM, which will restrict responses and therefore the score of certain items (e.g. response to the approaches of other children; appropriateness of social responses).

The most popular tool for the direct assessment of the child is the Autism Diagnostic Observation Schedule (ADOS) (Lord *et al.* 2000). Standardized activities and situations are presented to elicit communication, social interaction and imaginative play. The assessor looks out for any social communication deficits, fixated interests and repetitive behaviours which, if sufficiently severe when scored, would indicate a diagnosis of ASD. There are obvious drawbacks should the ADOS be used for a child already diagnosed or with a possible diagnosis of SM. Unable to communicate freely with an unfamiliar adult in an unfamiliar setting, the child would be likely to achieve a poor score and a possible misdiagnosis. It would be important to establish whether the parent felt the child's performance accurately portrayed his/her general interaction style, or if it was only typical of how he/she behaves with strangers.

Alternative or additional assessment tools

Given the difficulties of direct assessment of the child who is mute with strangers, the assessor would need to look for different ways to glean relevant information. If the child felt comfortable enough in a clinic room with close family members, observation might be possible through a one-way viewing mirror. Equally, a DVD of the child at home could be immensely helpful. In either case more weight might need to be given to the detailed parental interview, and to ensure that this information is supplemented by additional questionnaires or reports from any with whom the child communicates freely.

Probably the most important factor that needs accurate assessment when considering a possible ASD diagnosis is the question as to whether the child has empathy. Known previously as theory of mind, Simon Baron-Cohen (2003) describes it as 'the drive to identify another person's emotions and thoughts, and to respond to them with an appropriate emotion ... in order to connect or resonate with them emotionally.' Baron-Cohen states that 'ASD is primarily an empathy disorder'. So any measures or information about the presence or absence of empathy in a child, when with familiar people to whom she speaks comfortably, would be valuable.

Management of a child with SM and ASD (SM+ASD)

Keen *et al.* (2008) discovered that early identification and intervention are universally acknowledged as crucial for good management of SM. It follows that if any child has SM, regardless of any other diagnosis, it is still always important to address the SM as soon as possible. Yet sometimes people seem distracted by an additional diagnosis. For example, they might hasten to focus on teaching language skills to a child with additional language impairment, or social skills to a child who also has ASD, putting aside and sometimes contradicting intervention for SM. Consequently, the SM becomes more entrenched.

So, even if the child has SM+ASD, the SM must be addressed using methods that are known to be effective. The key ones are set out in Box 6.2 (see following page) and discussed with relevance to the dual diagnosis.

BOX 6.2 EFFECTIVE MANAGEMENT
OF SELECTIVE MUTISM

1. Early identification and intervention.

2. Education of all involved with the child about the nature of SM to ensure thorough understanding of the condition and united home/school team work.

3. Identification and adaptations of any factors that maintain the problem in order to create the right environment at home and school.

4. Acknowledgement and discussion of the difficulty with the child.

5. Introduction of informal small-step targets.

6. For older children, a specific coordinated behavioural programme of desensitization and graded exposure, such as stimulus fading (the 'sliding-in' technique).

7. Additional interventions, such as social skills, Cognitive Behaviour Therapy (CBT), or occasionally medication for older children and young people who present a more complex picture with co-morbid diagnoses.

In many ways the SM intervention need not be very different with the child with SM+ASD, provided that those involved have some understanding of ASD and knowledge of strategies that are helpful for the management of ASD. Nothing needs to change with regard to the first three items: early identification and intervention; education of all involved; and identification and adaptations of maintaining factors. When working directly with the child (items 4–6 in Box 6.2: acknowledgement and discussion of the difficulty; introducing informal small-step targets; and explaining a specific programme), additional visual support will be necessary to compensate for difficulties with abstract language and emotions. The small guide *Can I tell you about Selective Mutism?* (Johnson and Wintgens 2012), with its clear and simple information and line drawings, may be useful, and there is another in the series that describes ASD (Welton

2004). Stick men and simple line drawings or cartoons are helpful, as are facial expressions (graded smiling to sad faces) for a self-rated anxiety scale.

There are some other important considerations. Careful attention should be paid to finding suitable motivators for the SM+ASD child given their tendency not to be interested in more usual social rewards or reinforcers. Parents should have realistic expectations about the goals of SM therapy. With ASD there is a general reluctance to communicate, and the child is still likely to be non-communicative at times because they don't appreciate the need to be polite, or have natural curiosity in other people's affairs. In addition, all those involved with the child with SM+ASD will particularly need to be consistent and prepared for a long-term commitment to intervention.

Some autistic characteristics may impede progress with a specific SM programme, particularly sensory issues such as intolerance of noise or physical approaches. Likewise, the inability to use language outside the 'here-and-now' can make it hard to offer reassurance and hope when the child fails to progress or has a setback. However, it is possible to find ways round these factors, and once a specific co-ordinated behavioural programme of desensitization and graded exposure (such as stimulus fading, the 'sliding-in' technique) has been started, it is not uncommon to find that the rule-bound nature of a child with ASD is an advantage. The structure that the programme provides and the concrete rewards for each small step while progress is achieved give a feeling of safety and confidence. Soon, clear signs of an increased ability to speak out with more people in more situations can be observed.

CHAPTER 7

Selective Mutism and Stammering

Similarities and Differences

Jenny Packer

Stammering (also known as stuttering or dysfluency) and Selective Mutism (SM) are two different communication difficulties. Historically, it has been considered that the two conditions cannot co-occur: in fact, the *DSM-IV* (APA 1994) definition of SM highlights SM as a failure to speak in specific social situations, despite the ability to speak in other situations, not explained by another communication disorder. The exclusionary communication disorders are cited, and specifically include stammering. Evidence from clinical practice and discussions with colleagues working within both the fields of SM and stammering indicates, however, that the two conditions can and do co-occur. There has been little research into the co-occurrence of these two conditions, but information drawn from knowledge about both SM and stammering can be usefully compared.

Similarities between SM and stammering are numerous, and include factors relating to causality and onset, presentation, and management. With both SM and stammering there have been many different theories relating to causality, but up-to-date research within both areas suggests a genetic link in some cases. Modern theories also recognize multi-factorial causal and contributory features with both SM and stammering resulting from a variety of predisposing, precipitating and maintaining factors (see Kelman and Nicholas

2008 and Johnson and Wintgens 2001 for summaries of the different factors contributing to stammering and SM respectively, including genetic factors). The predisposing, precipitating and maintaining factors vary with each individual, but some commonalities are evident across the two conditions and can include temperamental traits, anxiety, reactions of others potentially reinforcing the condition, and avoidance of potentially distressing speaking situations acting to maintain the condition.

Other similarities relate to presentation: the potential for both SM and stammering to co-occur with other speech, language, cognitive or motor difficulties; typical age of onset; the variation in speech across different speaking situations; the fact that within both conditions more than just 'speech' is affected (with physical secondary behaviours such as loss of eye contact, facial grimacing or concomitant movements being part of stammering for some, and 'frozen' posture, lack of eye contact or facial expressions seen at times with SM); and that a continuum of severity is evident within both conditions.

Further similarities can be recognized in relation to the best ways to support both children with SM and those who stammer, with research showing early intervention to be effective for both conditions (Millard, Nicholas and Cook 2008; Johnson and Wintgens 2001). To enable this, full detailed assessment is recommended for both SM and stammering (Cline and Baldwin 2004; Guitar 2006), taking into account the individual's specific circumstances via information gained from parents, teachers and the child (as appropriate). Information should include: differences in speaking in different situations and environments; any coping strategies the child has developed; any known anxiety triggers; formal assessment of language skills as part of the assessment process (which may not be within the first meeting with the child). Non-directive play and rapport-building will likely play a part within the assessment for both a child who stammers and one presenting with SM in order to ensure the child does not feel under pressure that they 'must speak' during the assessment. Additionally, reassuring the child that they are not alone in finding it difficult to speak at times, and reducing any unintentional 'conspiracy of silence' about talking about the child's condition with them, can be a key part of assessment for both conditions.

Management approaches commonly used with SM and stammering following assessment show some overlap. Collaborative work with parents and school staff is important for effective management in both conditions, to ensure that a consistent approach is taken across different settings. In addition, instigating environmental changes to promote a relaxed communicative setting without direct pressure on the child's speaking is often part of early intervention for both conditions. More direct work often includes setting behavioural experiments in small steps and, for older children, principles of Cognitive Behavioural Therapy (Beck 1995) have been found to be effective with both stammering and SM.

The above examples show that there are a lot of similarities between SM and stammering; however, it is also important to recognize some clear differences between the two. Stammering has a much larger research base than SM alongside a wider prevalence: approximately 1 per cent in the general population (Bloodstein and Bernstein-Ratner 2007). Therapist confidence to work with SM may be less than seen with stammering, possibly reflecting the difference in the research and evidence bases between the two conditions. Another key difference between SM and stammering relates to gender, with stammering being more common in boys and SM more common in girls. Prognosis and relapse also differs – within SM it is generally recognized that once the condition has been successfully managed, relapse is not common, unlike in stammering where a cyclical pattern is freely acknowledged.

Both SM and stammering have many different presentations, and children who present with both stammering and SM do not all stammer in the same way, or present with the same pattern of mutism. Observations from clinical practice and information from discussions with other therapists show a variety of presentations. Both conditions can be evident at initial assessment; or the SM can develop after initial presentation of stammering, possibly due to embarrassment and consequent avoidance. It can be difficult in this circumstance to determine whether the child has developed SM or is showing extreme avoidance as part of their stammering presentation, but management would be similar in either case.

Possibly the most unexpected presentation is this: sometimes parents of children who initially present with SM report their child starting to stammer once the SM is resolving. Anecdotal evidence indicates that in these circumstances the stammer is typically characterized by part word and sound repetitions, usually at the start of utterances. Here a factor contributing to the onset of stammering may be the child's lack of experience of speaking within social situations, particularly with peers. Lack of practice with social skills such as turn-taking within conversations means that – when the child begins to feel comfortable to converse more – they experience time pressures speaking within social situations, so their turn to speak is 'marked' through repetitions at the start of their utterance while they process the rest of what they plan to say. Effective intervention should include acknowledging the stammer to reduce any anxiety the child associates with stammering, while working to develop social communication skills – for example, turn-taking and allowing the child to take the time to think about what they want to say before starting their conversational turn.

PART III

Interventions, Strategies and Supports

CHAPTER 8

Is Medication Helpful in Selective Mutism?

One Family's Experience and a Clinical Overview

Geoffrey Gibson and David Bramble

This chapter charts the progress of Simon (not his real name) in his journey to overcome Selective Mutism (SM). An attempt has been made to give as complete a picture as possible of the challenges faced by families raising a child with such special needs. It describes Simon's development of SM and how his family tried to come to terms with its effects and finally to find a way out of its more debilitating aspects. The broader issue of medication is also discussed.

Early years: birth to 2 years

Simon was born in 1996, the third child of a family that was, eventually, to grow to four with the arrival of a brother in 1997. Two older children were aged 12 and 9 at his birth. At the time Simon was born, the family lived and worked in Hungary as part of a teacher education scheme set up by the British Council. The older children were attending local primary schools and were completely bilingual. Both parents were fluent in Hungarian, though languages were kept reasonably distinct. The language of the home was English and that of school Hungarian. Simon was brought up speaking English and was surrounded, largely, by English-speaking people.

Simon's first two years were unremarkable. His mother looked after him at home. Having two older siblings ensured a lot of contact with other children. His early development followed a normal trajectory, although Simon was thought to have a much greater, and earlier, awareness of his surroundings than had been the case with his brother and sister. He seemed to be able to concentrate for longer, and more intently, than other children. At the age of two he would sit in front of Disney films for almost their entire duration without, apparently, getting distracted.

He was an early talker. At the time of John's birth he was already using multiple words and expressing himself clearly. In fact, his development of language seemed to be accelerated. It quickly became clear that the family as a whole needed to be careful what was said in his presence in case unwelcome repetitions occurred at inopportune moments. This is common for all parents, but what seemed to be different with Simon was his ability to focus on, and make some sense of, things that were going on around him but that were not specifically directed at him. On one occasion the family were watching a particularly bloody episode of *Casualty* on TV, when someone noticed that Simon had taken up distressed residence behind the sofa. For some years after this he would get hysterical at the sight of blood, particularly his own.

Trauma: age 2 years 4 months

Simon appeared to be a particularly sensitive person. One particular event stands out as a trigger for a whole raft of behaviours that would seem to directly lead to his SM.

The family holiday that year took them to the south of France and a meeting with three families, two of whom were seen regularly on trips home from Hungary. The other, the family of the father's brother, was seen less often. Since everyone was approaching the final destination from different directions it was agreed to meet at a campsite en route. Simon's family arrived first. The brother, who has a certain family resemblance to the father despite being three years younger, arrived a little later. They met up on one of the many campsite paths connecting tents and wash areas. Simon and his sister Jane (not her real name) had gone on ahead and came upon her uncle who had come looking for them. On seeing him, Simon ran into his arms and allowed himself to be thrown up in the air. It was only when he got a closer look that he realized the man who had hold of him was not his father but a strange man whom he did not know. He became hysterical and for the rest of the holiday (two weeks) lost his appetite and would not let any close member of the family out of his sight.

Pre-school, Hungary: ages 2 years 4 months to 4 years 4 months

On return to Hungary, Simon's mother was taking up a new six-month part-time appointment which entailed putting both Simon and John into a kindergarten. This is quite common in Hungary and facilities are generally excellent so there was no concern, even though he did not speak Hungarian. When the family had first arrived in Hungary the elder children had learned the language by doing this. However, Simon was different. He did not settle and made no effort to play with other children or speak the language.

It became clear that Simon had become increasingly agitated by the company of anyone who was not a close friend or family. If anyone visited the home, he would run away and hide, and if it was in the street, he would studiously avoid any sort of eye contact. It was not completely obvious that he had stopped talking altogether and, since a lot of friends were Hungarian, he could speak safely in the knowledge that it was only his family who could understand him.

However, it was on occasions when the family returned to the UK for family holidays that it became clear that Simon's difficulty in coping with anything out of the ordinary, particularly new people, was not normal, and not something that could simply be explained away by excessive shyness. The family would arrive home and it would take him at least two days before he would talk to his grandparents. Similarly, with each visit to close friends, it would take longer for him to settle in their company and engage in conversation. He stopped talking in the earshot of anyone with whom he was not familiar. Shopping was a nightmare, and fittings for new shoes nearly impossible.

The significance of this kind of behaviour was downplayed by the family, but there were times when it became impossible to ignore. On one occasion Simon got separated from the family and was discovered by a concerned passer-by. She explained that she had been at a loss to know what to do because she couldn't get any information about who he was and where his parents were.

Primary school, UK: ages 4 years 6 months to 5 years 6 months – SM in the school

The family returned to Britain full-time in 2001. Simon had gone to a number of kindergartens in Hungary but had not made any effort to interact with the other children. He would talk to his parents in front of other children and teachers at school but never to them directly, even if they spoke some English. It was not that he had never shown any desire to socialize with other children. He had made close friends with a number of English children and, having overcome his initial 'shyness' when returning home for holidays, he would happily join in games with children of close friends. Sadly, the problem turned out to be more serious than expected.

Simon started school at a small local primary school whose intake in the year that he joined was just four children. One of the boys joining the class – a boy called Chris – lived in the same village and appeared to have similar interests, although all attempts to introduce them to each other at village events over the preceding summer had met with failure. Simon had studiously rejected any suggestions of a get-together.

The task of taking him to school for the first time was left to his father. After lengthy discussions involving parents and the school it was felt that the presence of his mother might make it more, not less, difficult for him to get used to being left at school. Various methods at the different kindergartens he had gone to in Hungary had been tried (all of them involving staged withdrawal after varying lengths of time – some stretching to weeks). None of them had been particularly successful. Painful though it may be, it was decided this time to try the 'short sharp shock'. His father accompanied him into his classroom but quickly made excuses and left him with the teaching assistant and teacher, making it clear that there was always the telephone if he didn't calm down. He was picked up from school at the end of the day and the parents were told that Simon had cried solidly for nearly two hours. The school had been about to make contact when he calmed down enough to stop. He hadn't spoken to anyone at school but at this stage this wasn't the issue. After all, it was reasoned, he had been too upset to do so.

Over the next few weeks, Simon slowly improved when being left – that is to say he stopped crying – but he would not speak to anyone within the school environment. However, he did show some interest in getting to know Chris this time. On a trip to the local cinema he finally said something. His classmate's amazement was such that he didn't reply to Simon but looked at the rest of the family and said: 'Did you hear that? Did you hear that? Simon spoke.' After this Simon continued to speak to Chris outside of school and as long as he knew no one else from the school was listening. To a certain extent Chris became Simon's interpreter, being able to decipher the sign language and grunts that Simon used to communicate in the school playground. In the classroom it was different. Simon remained completely silent. As he learned to write he was given a white board and was able to write answers to class questions on this, but he would not speak.

Later, another child from Simon's class moved into the village and Simon was able to talk in front of her at home. The number of children Simon would speak to outside school rose to three, as new year groups joined Simon's, but this was where it stayed. Attempts were made to get Simon to speak to them on his own at school – when all the teachers and staff had gone – hoping that if he could hear his own voice at school when speaking in a non-threatening environment, he would be less 'afraid' of using it in front of others. Unfortunately, this never looked like becoming a useful strategy.

Obviously, Simon's behaviour caused considerable alarm both to his family and to the school. It wasn't long before steps were taken to seek medical intervention and consider issuing a statement of special needs in education. As anyone who has gone through this procedure will know, this is a very lengthy, bureaucratic and time-consuming business for parents. Eventually, Simon was referred both to the local educational psychologist and a child psychologist. After some time, Simon did feel able to speak in front of her. At least this enabled her to begin a diagnosis of his condition; above all, to establish whether his SM might be related to other problems of social anxiety or to investigate whether he might also fall on the autistic spectrum.

Simon's parents reported intense feelings of hopelessness. No one seemed to have had anything more than an incidental awareness of this kind of problem. Simon was referred to the Speech and Language Therapy department of the LEA and an advisor was appointed to work alongside Simon once a fortnight for an hour. At a loss to know how to proceed, the newly trained therapist asked the parents for advice. The suggestion was made of establishing a relationship through playing board games (in a separate room made available at the school). For the next year Simon was taken out of classes but there was no discernible improvement beyond an increased ability to succeed at card games: a wasteful indication that practitioner education in the matter of SM is essential.

Their sense of desperation at the lack of progress from the school and medical authorities eventually led the family to explore alternative treatment and research the condition more widely themselves. The following account is a breakdown of the different approaches that they tried during Simon's years at primary school. Most of these came about as a result of information provided by the charity Selective Mutism Information & Research Association (SMIRA), which was contacted after a search on the internet.

Primary school: ages 5 to 11
The work of Maggie Johnson and her co-author Alison Wintgens on a cognitive behavioural approach to the problem can be found in their

extremely practical *The Selective Mutism Resource Manual* (2001). This was bought by the school as a possible solution to the problems relating to Simon's treatment. In his second year both the school and the language therapist assigned to Simon tried to introduce some of the stimulus fading techniques – particularly the sliding-in approach. Sadly, there was no real success. It is difficult to decide whether this failed because of a lack of belief, a misunderstanding about how it should be implemented, or simply because in a small school it was impossible to invest in one child the amount of time and effort required for progress.

The child psychologist was very supportive of these efforts and, during the one-to-one therapy sessions, endeavoured to provide Simon with a mechanism to understand his emotions and quantify his fear of speaking on a scale of one to ten. Whilst this did help Simon confront his condition and give him some means to understand the way he was feeling, as far as allowing him to make practical progress in the school there appeared to be no substantive effect.

However, in the absence of any other obvious forms of treatment, a rather haphazard application of these techniques was tried out at the school, combined with regular – if rather infrequent – therapy sessions in the hospital. The latter were mainly geared towards establishing how far Simon could be categorized as belonging to the autistic spectrum.

At the school, Simon's silence was increasingly accepted as the norm. This meant that he could slip into the background during school work. He continued to use the white board to write answers on during class activities. For reading, the teachers had to rely on reports from the parents although, bizarrely, Simon would 'read to the teacher' by audibly mouthing words and indicating intonation patterns in sentences.

Socially, Simon wasn't exactly isolated. The other school children simply saw him as the child who doesn't talk. He wasn't excluded from playground games, but obviously his inability to communicate did not help integration. Periodically, a supply teacher would arrive and see his behaviour as deliberate defiance. On one occasion he was made to stand up in front of his classmates, while the teacher reprimanded him for not talking.

Treatment, during this period, consisted of the occasional initiative (such as personal white boards or pairing him with the one pupil he was known to speak to outside of class, Chris). His mother was also sometimes used as a supply teacher, having qualified as a primary teacher. None of these approaches seemed to have any noticeable effect. However, there were a few bright moments (whispering out of earshot, in a different room, to Chris) but nothing that could really qualify as a breakthrough or be regarded as lasting in any sense.

Ages 9 to 11: drug intervention – medication and its immediate aftermath

In the face of this lack of progress, and aware that his condition was likely to be an increasing problem for his educational development beyond primary school, his parents applied themselves to researching alternative forms of treatment. One approach that seemed to be shunned in the UK, but which was common practice in the USA, was the use of anti-depressant drugs and in particular the use of fluoxetine (commonly known by its trade name, Prozac). It was thus timely when a TV company approached SMIRA for volunteers on a documentary they were seeking to do on SM. They explained that they were looking to follow two children through a course of treatment: one taking the behavioural therapy route, the other medication. Simon was keen to be involved, partly because he recognized the kudos of being filmed for TV and partly because he saw medication as a possible magic bullet, solving all his problems in one go (RDF Media – Help me to Speak 2006).

A request was made to his psychologist to see whether such treatment might be tried out in his case. Whilst not being a particular supporter of the medication route, his psychologist felt that in this case, especially since Simon was enthusiastic to try it, there was merit in giving it a go as long as it was properly supervised by a trained psychiatrist whom she had already identified.

The involvement of the TV company was also considered important since it was clear that Simon saw this as having high cachet value as far as his peers were concerned. The hope was that it would boost his self-esteem as much as the medication would. The filming was a very low-key affair with only two people involved in interviewing and camera work. They worked hard to establish a relationship with Simon, and interviewed family and professionals (both educational and medical) to get a picture of how the condition had affected all concerned. Simon responded well and was prepared to talk, however minimally, about his feelings on camera. Filming at school illustrated the extent of his problems and the various coping mechanisms he, his classmates and the school used to try and overcome communication difficulties. There was a particularly revealing moment when Simon explained how he felt when being surprised by someone he identified with school at a church event where he was talking normally. 'As soon as I saw him, I felt as though I had been betrayed.' That he had somehow violated his personal space.

The treatment with fluoxetine began after an initial consultation with the psychiatrist and an explanation of the possible side-effects and risks. On the kind of low dosage that would be used with an eight-year-old these were not particularly frightening. Treatment would begin with a daily dose of 2.5ml which would be increased to 5ml gradually unless there were unpleasant reactions. The theory was that since fluoxetine increases the uptake of naturally produced serotonin, the drug can help to reduce inhibition in children.

The results, whilst not spectacular, were noticeable. Simon seemed to be visibly more relaxed when approached by strangers. He overcame his reluctance to speak to shop assistants and did not hide when visitors came to the house. He was much more care-free, less reticent, when playing games with Chris. However, at school there was little change, though perhaps more willingness to communicate through signing and a greater desire to join in playground football games. Indeed, one of the supply teachers tried to take advantage of this by making him captain of the school football team for one match. As an interview in the film demonstrates, this provoked an acknowledgement of how important verbal communication is on the football field, but also an insight into how (in his own mind) he was able to overcome it by a complicated series of hand signals. As far as classroom work was concerned, he remained locked in silence.

The most dramatic result of the treatment came after approximately six months when the parents encouraged him to invite a group of school friends around for his birthday party which would consist of a game of five-a-side football. Amongst those invited were at least three children who he had never spoken in front of. The day came and, true to his word, as soon as he opened the door on them, he began speaking as though there had never been an issue. On the football field, for the first time he was able to shout 'pass, shoot, give it to me, tackle' where before he had simply mouthed the words. There was a clear feeling of liberation, and as far as these children were concerned – as long as they were nowhere near the school – he was no longer affected by SM when he was with them after this day. However, the school remained a major sticking point. He wouldn't talk on the school premises.

Simon carried on taking the fluoxetine, under supervision, with regular (monthly) sessions with the psychiatrist until the start of the summer holidays (in total for around nine months), when he decided that he would like to give it a rest for a while.

He declined to go back on it when he returned to school after the summer holiday. To a certain extent, this would be a litmus test for the long-term effect that the drug (or the accompanying film) had had on his condition.

There was no doubt that he was much more confident at school, although perhaps this was a result of seniority. Simon was now in Year 6. He still did not speak in class but there were rare occasions when he was observed to whisper something in the playground to his group of friends. This situation remained for the rest of his time at primary school.

However, there were some major developments in other areas. At the beginning of the new school year his mother was able to spend a little more time at the school. She would go into class and take out a group of children to do work on a group and individual level. The idea was to select children who Simon had spoken to outside of school in the hope that they would make him feel more comfortable. At first it didn't seem to help, but after about four weeks Simon began to speak and by the end of this period he was even having to be told to shut up. Whilst, as mentioned above, this did not translate to the rest of the school, it was still a significant development which demonstrated to him that speaking in the school environment was possible after all.

This was particularly important since he was in the process of choosing his secondary school and it was clear that his initial reaction to that school would play a big role in determining whether he carried his SM with him or left it at the gates of his primary school. There were a number of factors that seemed crucial as far as this decision was concerned. He didn't want to go to a school where a lot of his fellow classmates would be going. He had set his sights on going to a school which one of his best friends already attended. His parents arranged a meeting with the Head Teacher and head of year, to plan a staged transition for him. It appears that at this meeting Simon managed to speak to the Head in his office. He was also able to speak when attending the various introductory days organized for new pupils at the school.

Outside of the school environment he had also become more confident. He was able to speak to the vicar during Confirmation classes, even though there were other children (from different primary schools) present during these sessions.

The fact that all of these developments came about after he had stopped his treatment with fluoxetine suggests that the gains made while on it – confidence and assurance – were not completely lost. That does not mean to say there were not any setbacks. At football practice one morning he phoned home, in some distress, to ask to be fetched early. He appears to have had some sort of panic attack triggered by feeling sick. The same thing happened at a local Valentine's Day party when his favourite song was played over the sound system.

Secondary school: ages 11 to 15

Overall, the transition to secondary school and his ability to take part in lessons was remarkably painless given the difficulties he had experienced with all other starts in his education. The fact that he was going to a school of his choice with people he wanted to be with, and having made a conscious decision that it was going to be different, seems to have emboldened him. Whilst he will never come across as the most garrulous of students, he can at least function in a modern communicative classroom. This ability, however, perhaps disguises some more lasting issues that it is easy to overlook when one sees how far he has come.

He still is prone to panic attacks. These seem to manifest themselves when he feels he is unable to control his emotions, or be in control of events. For example, a visit to the York dungeons with a friend resulted in him having to leave; a trip to a local football match where a seat behind a goal left him feeling vulnerable to misdirected shots; going to parties where he might not know everyone. He has a tendency to get rather obsessed by certain things, or routines.

Set against this there are numerous successes. His ability to focus has turned him into a very good drummer and he even played in a band at his sister's wedding. He has been on a variety of school trips with no problems. He has a good circle of friends and seems to be able to fit in with his peer group. For example, he doesn't ever seem to have been affected by bullying. He can now talk to his teachers in class. Those who have no knowledge of his past find it difficult to believe that he didn't speak at all in primary school.

There is no doubt that Simon has been on a very definite journey with his SM. It is difficult to say whether it has been completely conquered or removed. It is more that, as he has grown, he has been able to develop certain coping mechanisms that allow him to function in society. There are circumstances when his natural reaction is to try to avoid unsettling situations. This can make him over-cautious and, in a school environment, retiring. However, if the rewards are there for him, he has a clear determination to make sure that he can reach them.

The role of fluoxetine

On the face of it there seems little doubt that the decision to try fluoxetine to reduce his anxiety was the right one. As Maggie Johnson has said, it should never be seen as a complete panacea, but it can help to create the conditions where progress can begin to be made. Simon had no real side-effects from the drug apart from occasional sweatiness at night, and he only ever took small doses – 5ml was the maximum. It didn't seem to deaden emotions in the way that other users sometimes describe. If anything, the tendency to lessen inhibitions meant that it was necessary for his parents to keep a watchful eye on over-boisterous behaviour. As Simon said, it seemed to give him a window onto a world free from the paralyzing constraints of social anxiety.

However, important as fluoxetine was, the whole experience of being filmed for TV and being the centre of attention in a non-threatening way was equally significant. This enabled him to be more comfortable in himself, which in turn has allowed him to open out and express himself.

Conclusion

Simon has now reached the stage where his SM – in its severe form – is largely confined to the past. He can cope with strangers at home and outside. He remains undemonstrative and certainly too self-aware for his own good, but he is learning to exercise some control over the anxiety levels which enforce this. It is important to keep an open mind about the effect his medication had on his journey, but there is no denying that it coincided with a gradual improvement in his condition. Above all, it would appear to be a valuable addition to the full range of treatment that is available to sufferers of SM. Simon's example, and the journey his family have been through as a result of it, is surely a testament to the need for flexibility in the face of a condition that is, in itself, so inflexible.

Comment

The remainder of this chapter has been contributed by Dr David Bramble, in his capacity as a child psychiatrist.

This account of Simon's life to date illustrates perfectly the challenge posed to families and health, educational and other specialist professionals when confronted by such case-complexity. After what appears to be two years of essentially normal development, Simon changed, and his habitual communication and social interactive styles particularly so. These concerns were picked up, as is usually the case, first by his parents and were shared by the nursery staff and his first teachers subsequently. The picture of articulate, middle-class parents seemingly moving heaven and earth in order to make full use of what resources were available to get to the bottom of their son's difficulties and then address them really early on in his life is very familiar to clinicians working in the fields of neurodisability and paediatric mental health. In Simon's case, his extremely handicapping shyness and highly selective communicative style were also associated with marked situational anxiety (which occasionally progressed to full-blown panic attacks) as well as some features suggestive of accompanying autistic traits, but the results of any subsequent investigation or help on this score are not presented.

From the perspective of medical treatment, the fact that the boy was evidently experiencing severe and handicapping degrees of anxiety was acknowledged and the environmental, educational and behavioural management strategies available for him were attempted before medication was considered. This general approach, with a few exceptions, is axiomatic in modern paediatric mental health practice and particularly when helping children with anxiety-related disorders. However, when these approaches were found wanting, the selection of a form of medication that is regarded as a standard treatment for chronic anxiety in older adolescents and adults was prescribed, and to good effect. Sometimes, in order to bring about symptomatic relief rapidly before the fluoxetine normally begins to work (four to six weeks) another type of medication, diazepam, may be used.

Simon took fluoxetine for nine months in his late childhood and it was acknowledged that it was more than likely that this specifically helped him make a step-change in terms of mastering his SM symptoms by relieving his situational anxiety and enhancing his confidence, notwithstanding his evidently relished novel role as the subject of a television programme! These benefits were accrued without the troublesome side-effects that are often experienced when this form of treatment is prescribed. Medication, when used in this way, commonly complements other therapeutic and special educational measures.

Despite not taking fluoxetine over the period, Simon's transition to secondary school went reasonably well even though this represents a period of heightened anxiety and uncertainty for many anxiety-prone children and particularly so for autistic children. It was interesting to note that Simon's confidence and ability to communicate clearly and authoritatively was reportedly particularly evident whilst he was playing football, and serves to emphasize how team-based exercise coupled with a sense of shared purpose (i.e. sport) can temporarily override inhibiting degrees of anxiety. Physical fitness per se is very important in promoting confidence in children with anxiety-related problems.

General information on medication and SM

Whilst defined as a distinct anxiety-based disorder in the latest editions of the major disease classification systems, SM may be seen to represent a relatively uncommon 'final common pathway' of expression of a range of paediatric mental health and developmental problems and also commonly overlaps with several other discrete conditions where handicapping anxiety and social phobia are prominent (Kopp and Gillberg 1997; Kristensen 2000). This heterogeneity of aetiologies (causes) and associations will help explain why, to date, no large-scale controlled clinical trials of any form of drug treatment have been conducted specifically for SM. Rather, the extant literature rests upon small studies involving single cases, case series (Carlson et al. 1999) and small controlled studies of patients with SM whose handicapping anxieties were sufficiently severe and unresponsive to other measures as to merit a trial of drug therapy (Black and Uhde 1994). Nevertheless, what is emerging from this is the wider recognition that classes of drug that relieve handicapping anxiety tend to work best in helping patients with SM master their situationally specific social communication difficulties.

It is axiomatic in British child mental health practice that treatment is very rarely primarily drug-based; rather, targeted medication is best applied as part of an integrated, multi-modal therapeutic package which is tailored to the needs of individual children. Furthermore, in potentially long-term conditions such as SM, as the child matures such treatment commonly has to be adjusted to meet changing needs.

Modern clinical practice also requires that formal 'care plans' are elaborated in order to ensure that everyone involved in the child's care knows what their roles are and what individual objectives they have to work towards so as to avoid any potential confusion or duplication of effort.

So in the case of SM where non-pharmacological, psychological, speech and language therapy and educational measures are either not working or are only partially effective through the presence of handicapping degrees of anxiety for any given individual, and after specific anxiety-reducing psychological therapies (such as relaxation and cognitive behavioural therapy) have been tried, consideration of anxiety-reducing medication is commonly the next step. It must be emphasized that drug therapy is not always necessary and tends to be reserved for older children and adolescents, and those with more severe and pervasive difficulties – that is, difficulty speaking in all major life settings – and those with handicapping associated mental health difficulties, or 'co-morbidities', such as depression, panic disorder and obsessive compulsive disorder. Furthermore, the child who is also autistic tends to require more physical treatment of this sort.

Types of medication

Modern paediatric psychopharmacology now has a wide range of agents to draw from, but in the case of treating handicapping anxiety two broad classes are used in everyday practice: benzodiazepines and selective serotonin re-uptake inhibitors (SSRIs).

1. *Benzodiazepines.* The most common agent used in this group is diazepam ('Valium'), which has been available for 50 years; another popular drug in this class is lorazepam. These agents provide rapid reduction in anxiety by enhancing the action of a brain chemical called GABA. In short-term use they are generally safe and effective and work quickly (within an hour of ingestion) but are not recommended for long-term use because they can produce tolerance (i.e. higher doses required to produce the desired effect) and dependence (i.e. a need to continue to avoid unpleasant withdrawal symptoms); this is why it is recommended that they are used only for a few weeks if taken regularly (i.e. every day). Most commonly, they are prescribed to be used on an intermittent basis and in anticipation of particularly anxiety-provoking situations (e.g. exam vivas, public speaking, acting or singing performances) or as a temporary measure on a regular daily basis before SSRIs start working in patients experiencing chronic and handicapping anxiety (see next section). Whilst generally regarded as being a rather safe medication, benzodiazepines can, very occasionally, produce paradoxical effects which include irresponsible behaviour, aggression or even delirium (a temporary confusional state). Another important consideration when using this class of drug is that they are known to inhibit learning through interference with memory formation; therefore, if taken for longer periods they may counter or interfere with remedial educational or psychotherapeutic measures the child is also receiving. Patients with breathing difficulties such as sleep apnoea and chronic bronchitis should not take these drugs because they can potentially severely aggravate these conditions. Dosages are usually low (1 to 2mg twice to three times a day) and a

liquid version is also available. For situational anxiety, higher single doses may be required. It is recommended that patients do not take this medication regularly for more than four to six weeks.

2. *SSRIs.* A particularly well-known example of this class of agent is fluoxetine hydrochloride ('Prozac'); whilst it was developed 40 years ago to be a safe and effective anti-depressant medication and is now the most commonly prescribed drug for this condition in the world, subsequent research and clinical experience has demonstrated that it is also a very effective means of treating generalized and chronic anxiety. However, unlike the benzodiazepines, this treatment usually takes several weeks to exert its therapeutic effects (normally 6–8 weeks) and can produce more, although mostly mild, side-effects. SSRIs are generally alerting (or wakefulness-promoting) drugs; therefore, they tend to be taken as a single dose in the morning. They have a long duration of action so that an occasional missed dose will normally not be noticed in terms of a rapid return of anxiety, and sometimes they are taken every other day. Whilst precisely how they exert their anxiety-reducing effect is not fully understood, they are known to boost the brain chemical serotonin which is the principal moderator of mood in certain parts of the brain and also promote the growth of mood-enhancing brain cells in specific brain areas such as the hippocampus. Fluoxetine is generally well tolerated, although mild side-effects such as nausea, blurred vision, constipation or diarrhoea are relatively common but short-lived; in older patients the drug is known to reduce sex drive and can induce insomnia. The latter condition may be prevented by giving the drug as a single dose in the morning (the usual regimen). Commonly employed dosages are 20 to 40mg a day, although lower initial doses are used with younger patients and higher doses in older patients particularly where obsessional and compulsive symptoms are also prominent. A typical trial of this treatment is two to three months and, if shown to be both effective and well tolerated (i.e. not producing uncomfortable

serious side-effects) by this time, then it is continued up to six months at which point, and if there isn't a pressing reason not to, a staged withdrawal over a month is undertaken to test ongoing need. Should the handicapping anxiety return and if all other non-drug supportive measures remain in place, then the drug is recommenced and taken for another year. Over this time the child should be reviewed every few months to check compliance, emergence of side-effects or for dose adjustment. Other drugs in this class are citalopram and sertraline, which may be substituted for fluoxetine.

Antihistamines and buspirone may be used in a similar, short-term or prophylactic way as diazepam. The anti-depressant drug venlafaxine that enhances the effects of both serotonin and noradrenaline in the brain may be used as a long-term treatment when the SSRIs prove ineffective. The anti-epilepsy drug pregabalin is also used as a second-choice treatment of generalized anxiety in adults but has not been studied in children or adolescents for this indication.

Other considerations

Whilst a particular medication might appear objectively entirely suitable for a particular patient, there may be resistance to taking it encountered from the family and the child. These considerations should be addressed in a sensitive manner and it may take a while to gain the trust required to try it. There are also families where a wait-and-see approach is appropriate because rapid changes in symptoms can occur over a modest time period. Some people may not be able to swallow tablets or do not tolerate the taste of particular liquid forms of the chosen drug, so awareness of alternative preparations (such as taste-neutral drops) may be preferred. Any patient taking medication for mental heath problems should be reviewed regularly (but not necessarily frequently) and screened for compliance, treatment response and emerging side-effects.

Summary

Whilst medication does not 'cure' SM, it can significantly relieve the associated anxiety and also ameliorate other co-morbidities so as to help 'jump start' children to begin to gain greater benefit from psycho-educational measures which are commonly used to treat the condition. Any trial of medication should be under the supervision of a clinician with appropriate experience of both SM and paediatric psychopharmacology who is also prepared to work collaboratively with all other professionals involved in a given case and also ensure that any other co-morbidities present are also addressed satisfactorily.

CHAPTER 9

Successful Approaches to Selective Mutism in School and Community Settings

Jyoti Sharma, Jane Kay, Susan Johnson and Rae Smith

As explained in Chapters 1 and 2, some 'predisposing factors' for Selective Mutism (SM) (such as children's temperament) and 'precipitating factors' (such as fright on entering nursery) are hard to avoid, but what have been called 'maintaining factors' such as the attitudes and behaviour of people around the children can be altered to good effect. Some of the ways in which SM has been successfully challenged will be explored in this chapter.

Using a Play Interaction approach to help children with SM

Our first example has been provided by Jyoti Sharma, a play interaction specialist working in the Leicester City Autism Outreach Service. Fortunately, she and her colleagues are encouraged to provide assistance to some SM children who do not have a diagnosis of autism, but who fail to communicate at school. Notable features of this team's approach are the absence of criticism of the children and a gentle use of humour, non-verbal support and low-level technological assistance.

Introduction

The Play Interaction Programme has been running for over ten years, working with a wide range of children and young people with SEN (Special Educational Needs), including those with autism, ADHD, sensory impairments and social/emotional difficulties.

In my work as a Play Interaction Specialist I have found this approach to be effective for children described as having SM, enabling them to become more confident and comfortable with social interaction and communication in school.

What is Play Interaction?

The Play Interaction Programme is a bespoke Leicester City training programme for teaching assistants within primary schools. It incorporates a range of interactive strategies to help develop children's social interaction and communication skills through a play-based approach, drawing on techniques used in approaches such as drama, art work, 'Treatment and Education of Autistic and related Communication Handicapped Children' (TEACCH) (Schopler 1997), Intensive Interaction (Nind and Hewett 1994/1996/2001), Music Interaction (Prevezer 1990) and Laban Movement (Preston-Dunlop 1998).

The Play Interaction Programme began in 2000. Its goal was to train staff in school to meet the needs of pupils with social communication and interaction difficulties. Over these ten years the programme has been consolidated into a taught package and manual. Follow-up support is provided to schools that have accessed the full training. This includes opportunities for staff to share ideas and information through networks and briefings.

The Programme and structure of sessions

To initiate training in the Play Interaction Programme, schools have to apply via a member of the Special Needs Teaching Service. The application request includes the needs of a 'target child' and any interventions currently being used to meet that child's needs. The Programme is designed to meet the needs of that particular child, although a parallel aim is to cascade the broader skills of how to teach/support social communication and interaction via the 'target child's' programme.

Initially a meeting is held with the parent/carer, the school and any other key adults. This is a fact-finding meeting to ascertain the child's strengths and interests, as well as their needs. From this meeting and an observation of the child, a programme is written based on the format in our Play Interaction Manual.

The sessions ideally take place in a distraction-free room, once a week for approximately 30 to 45 minutes for up to ten weeks. The programme is then reviewed with parents/carers and school staff members.

Each session is structured and planned according to the needs of the child. Visual structure and communication support is used, for example: a visual timetable, choice boards, 'Yes' and 'No' cards and communication symbols. These visual cues help the individual child to reduce levels of anxiety and enable them to know what is expected in the session.

A session usually starts with a 'Meet and Greet' activity. This is then followed by two play activities and then a choice of activity as a reward. It ends with a 'Goodbye' activity. The programme is initially child-centred, consisting of the adult following the child's lead through imitating the child's actions and sharing the child's interests. This often includes the child's playing or engaging in his or her favoured activities a number of times before adult-directed activities are introduced. Once the child is ready, familiar peers are invited in as sociable buddies. This is done with the child's permission. When appropriate, the sessions are generalized with familiar people/ peers in other social settings – for example, in the corridor, in the playground and classroom. It should be noted that all of this is done at the child's pace.

Case study

When Nina (not her real name) was referred to me for Play Interaction I had been running the programme successfully for ten years but had little experience of working with pupils with SM. I recognized that I would need to rapidly increase my own awareness and understanding of SM. I turned to the following books: *Silent Children* by Rosemary Sage and Alice Sluckin (2004) and *The Selective Mutism Resource Manual* by Maggie Johnson and Alison Wintgens (2001). At the time of intervention Nina was eight years old and in Year 5 in a mainstream city primary school. I observed her in the classroom. She did not speak to her peers or adults. She responded to the questions of others by using hand gestures and facial expressions. However, when playing in the playground I heard her speak to one of her peers, but when I moved closer to her she stopped talking. Nina's mother reported that at home she spoke to her family members in clear Gujarati sentences and was able to understand complex language. She was described as a 'chatterbox' at home. School reported that they had long-standing concerns about Nina not speaking to adults and her peers in the classroom. For instance, she would not respond to her name during registration time.

SESSION 1

A couple of days after my observation, I collected Nina from the classroom. She lowered her head and walked stiffly with me to the room. When we got to the room I greeted her and explained that I would be coming to play some games with her. She did not make any eye contact with me.

I used this session to try to form a trusting relationship with Nina. I understood that SM children become very anxious in social situations. In order to help reduce her anxieties I showed her a list of printed activities on the wipe board that we were going to do together, a lot of which involved her making a choice. She agreed to mark a tick next to each printed activity as she completed it. This visual structure was used in the hope of reducing her anxieties within the session, enabling her to know what was expected and how long the session would last.

During 'Meet and Greet' I showed her some emotion picture cards: 'Happy', 'Sad' and 'Angry'. I pointed to the 'Happy' picture card to express how I was feeling today. When I asked how she was feeling, she also pointed to the 'Happy' picture card but her facial expression did not display this emotion.

I gave Nina the opportunity to choose a game to play from a choice of two games. She made no response to make her choice known to me. In the end I chose 'Stack 'em Up' and she nodded her head when I asked for her approval.

To see how she would respond to me I made some deliberate mistakes. I called her by a different name, and she smiled at this. I then deliberately took her turn in the game; she looked at me and giggled.

In order to discover Nina's interests, I drew on a piece of paper a spider web of things she might like to play and she wrote down 'colouring' and 'hide and seek'. She later chose to do a drawing of a butterfly; I also drew a butterfly on my piece of paper alongside her. I praised her drawing and during this process I commented on the things that I like to do and asked her if she also liked doing the same. She responded to the questions by pointing to the 'Yes' and 'No' cards, which were placed on the table.

SESSION 2

Nina's responses in the next session were the same as in Session 1. Again she chose to do a drawing of a butterfly. I asked her if she wanted to invite a friend in the next session. She nodded her head and then wrote her friend's name down on the wipe board. She chose the friend she spoke to in the playground. She made brief eye contact with me and smiled when I agreed to this.

SESSION 3

When having her peer in the session, Nina's body posture appeared very relaxed and not stiff as noted in the previous sessions. She was given the written checklist in order to show her peer what we were going to play in the session. During the 'Meet and Greet' slot in the session, when focusing on feelings Nina surprised me when she whispered 'I am happy' in her peer's ear in response to her peer's question 'How are you feeling today?'

She actively participated in the miming game 'Change the Stick' (a game consisting of a person pretending the stick to be something else by using mimes and others having to guess what it may be). She used mimes to pretend the stick was a spoon and later a lipstick. I heard her laugh for the first time at her peer when she got her answer wrong in the game.

Nina later made some 'h' sounds when using the BIGmack (a voice recording device) and enjoyed playing it back. She began to write and draw her responses on a piece of paper. She later managed to do the same within the classroom. In addition, she used the 'Yes' and 'No' cards in response to being asked closed questions. She was sometimes heard to whisper her answers in a friend's ear.

SESSIONS 4 AND 5

In session 4, we made sound conversation on the mobile phones and on the BIGmack. She enjoyed going out of the room with her peer and listening to a message being recorded on the device. They then brought it back into the room and played it back to me. I had to guess whose voice it was and sometimes I deliberately made a wrong guess. This made her laugh and she pointed to the 'No' card. On another occasion the two girls went out of the room to record a voice; they later came back and played the voice to me. To my surprise it was Nina's voice being recorded! She recorded a quiet 'Hello' for me to hear. At this point she pointed to herself and smiled. I was truly amazed at this breakthrough! She actually wanted me to hear her voice! In session 5 she said 'Hello' to me on the phone.

SESSIONS 6 AND 7

I asked Nina if she would like to hear my friend say 'Hello' on the mobile. She made a sound, which I took as a 'Yes'. At this point a new adult said 'Hello' to her on the mobile from outside of the room. To my surprise she said 'Hello' back to the adult. This adult was gradually introduced into the session, though initially from a distance and not engaging in the games.

The girls later engaged in the same miming activity; during this time the adult moved closer to the girls while they engaged in pretend play. Nina began to give one-word responses to identify what the person was pretending the stick to be. She gave quick glances at the adult coming closer; fortunately, this did not faze her. In session 7 she was able to continue engaging and using single-word responses while the adult was sitting within the group.

SESSIONS 8 TO 10

In session 8 Nina took control of the written activities checklist, reading them out to the others. I nearly fell off my chair with surprise!

When it was her turn to share her feelings during the 'Meet and Greet' in the session, she pointed to the angry emotion picture card and said, 'I'm angry because you were late to bring me here!' When her peer asked her about her weekend, she replied, 'It was a normal day.'

Later, when someone shouted out the answer in one of the games, she said, 'Put your hand up.'

When playing with the puppets, she progressed from just handling the puppets to gradually making some quiet sounds for the puppets and then to eventually saying, 'The little boy (boy puppet) can be the doctor in the story.' She put on a voice for the puppet as she handled it. She said, 'I am the doctor, now what can I do for you?'

When doing a shared drawing with the others, she went from just quietly drawing butterflies and making patterns to answering my question about what she was drawing. She said, 'It's a butterfly, a happy one because it is colourful and has stripes.'

At this point two more of her chosen friends were invited in the session. We played the game 'I went to the shop and bought a…'. On her turn she said, 'I went to the shop and bought my brother' and then she laughed.

I later explained to the children that we were going to play our miming pretend game in the communal hall because someone else needed to use the room. When carrying out the same activity in another setting, to my surprise Nina continued talking to her peers and adults while other people were passing by her. This was a considerable step forward for her.

In session 10 Nina began to interrupt others talking and at this point we had to introduce the visual group rules for listening and taking turns when others were speaking!

MEMBERS OF STAFF REPORT ON NINA'S FOLLOW-UP PROGRESS

The teacher reported that since the programme Nina was beginning to answer to her name being called out during registration time; she used a normal volume of speech. The teacher also heard her speak to other members of staff on duty in the playground; she initiated a conversation with a variety of adults and peers. On one occasion she commented on how she didn't have anything spotty to wear for 'Children in Need day'.

I carried out a follow-up meeting with the SEN teacher on 21 May 2013 to find out whether Nina had continued to speak. The teacher said, 'We are delighted with the change in Nina. I teach her on Wednesdays so I have been able to witness it firsthand, which has been great. She continues to talk to her peers and to adults. In fact I joked with her the other day when I was on dinner duty – there was such a noise over the general noise of lunchtime that I turned round to ask the culprit to be quieter, and it was Nina. I did say to myself that I never thought I would be asking her to make less noise. Nina laughed with me. Nina takes part in class discussions and puts her hand up to make useful contributions, she really is a part of everything now. In terms of social interaction she really is one of the girls who has got a good group of friends. She is doing well academically. She makes significant contributions in group work; even when she is working with a very confident, strong-minded friend who could easily overshadow her.'

Further follow-up, however, revealed a different story. After a full term in her new secondary school, although Nina had been observed speaking briefly to peers in the playground, she had not spoken to a single member of staff. Ongoing support and preparation for her transfer had clearly been needed. Fortunately, it will now be possible to brief the senior school staff about SM and undertake some more work with Nina herself.

Snapshots of two other case studies

I implemented the same visual structure and communication support within the sessions with two other children. At the time of intervention Josh (not his real name) was aged eight and was in a Year 3 class in a mainstream primary school. Members of school staff reported long-standing concerns about him not speaking in school. However, his parents reported that he spoke fluently and confidently in the home setting with all his family members in English. It took over eight sessions for Josh to start speaking with two peers and three adults during the sessions. He responded to adults sharing his interest in football. Opportunities were given to him to be in charge of the written activities checklist. He relaxed and laughed when I teased him when hiding the ball. He found it funny that I needed reminders to kick the ball and not hold it in my arms when playing football; this enabled him to use some gestures and later one-word responses to correct my deliberate mistakes when playing the game.

He progressed from making sounds in an echoing microphone and voice recorder to saying single words and short phrases to using sentences. The class teacher and the TA (teaching assistant) both reported that he is now using a normal volume and tone of voice within the classroom. He has also put up his hand to volunteer to engage in role-playing in the Christmas Play. During the session he said, 'I'm happy because I'm here to play.' I recall him in the initial sessions having been reluctant and shy when trying out new activities but during the later sessions in the programme his confidence grew.

I also worked with Neha (not her real name) who was in Year 1 in mainstream primary school. Her teacher reported that she had not heard Neha speak at all. The teacher reported how difficult it was to assess Neha's ability levels in different areas of learning as she did not share her thoughts and views and she would not read aloud. It was also reported that Neha did not participate in the play of others. However, her parents reported that she spoke fluently in Gujarati and in English in the home setting with her family members.

During my intervention a significant turning point was noted when Neha recorded her own voice on her father's mobile at home while reading a storybook to her dolls (this was a suggestion that I had made to her parent). The parent shared the voice recording with the class teacher in front of Neha. The teacher praised and rewarded Neha for good reading and said what a delight it was to hear her voice. The parent mentioned that Neha had asked him to record her voice again while she read a story to her dolls so that the teacher could hear her voice on the recorder again. This demonstrated that Neha wanted the teacher to hear her voice.

Conclusion

The Play Interaction approach provided the children with a relaxed, fun and motivating environment, free from direct demands or pressures to speak. Using individual children's interests such as football and drawing enabled me to build a trusting relationship with them. I was able to present myself as an equal play buddy. The sessions provided the individual children with opportunities to relate to others in their own time and at their own pace.

I found that incorporating a sense of humour and making deliberate mistakes enabled the children to take on a lead role in order to correct my mistakes. This technique helped boost self-confidence and self-esteem. The gradual inviting of the target child's peers and adults was similar to the 'sliding-in' and the 'fading-in' techniques (Johnson and Wintgens 2001). Using activities such as 'When I went to the shop...' reflected 'The Talking Circle' approach used in the SM manual (Johnson and Wintgens 2001).

Crucially, several factors within the sessions successfully helped reduce anxiety levels in the children. These included the use of visual structures, playfulness and humour, and non-directive play approaches using puppets and toys of particular interest to the children.

According to Sage and Sluckin (2004), 'the most common reason for a child's failure to speak is said to be anxiety' (p.7).

Working with a young man to promote social development and employment

Next, we hear from Jane Kay who is employed as a 'Connexions' worker to ensure that young people do not disappear into permanent exclusion from society. At the time of publication this service still exists, though with reduced funding and a reduction in what appears to have been a fairly generous time allocation.

Again, the approach involves a trusting relationship, non-verbal support and incorporation of technology.

During the time of this case study I was employed as a Connexions Personal Adviser working intensively with young people who had multiple barriers preventing them from entering employment, education or training. My aim was to support young people by helping them work through their issues and eventually move into training, work or education.

I first met William (not his real name) when he was 18 and due to leave school in the summer of 2002. He was referred to me by a Personal Adviser who specialized in Careers Guidance. He did not speak at school, apart from the odd word to one member of staff. He comes from a large family but spoke very little at home and only to his mother and very young brother. He had stayed on at school as there wasn't really an alternative for him at the time, but had spent most of his time working alone in a resource room. Our first meeting took place in school just after Easter of that year. William nodded and shook his head appropriately in answer to questions I asked him. I had gathered as much information as I could about him from the referring Personal Adviser, his mother and the special educational needs teacher at school. From this I learnt that he was interested in computers and reading; from questioning William himself, I found out that he held a provisional driver's licence but had not had any lessons. I was aware of his capabilities from the school statements and also noticed fairly soon that William had an excellent sense of humour.

As a first step, I took my laptop into school along with a CD-ROM which replicates the theory driving test. We managed to undertake this test by me reading out the text from the screen and William nodding at the answer he felt was correct. From this we gathered that William was more than ready to take to the roads, but I myself, who had been driving for over 25 years, should be banished from them immediately!

When the end of term came and he left school, William agreed that I could come to visit him at his home. I didn't want him to get used to the idea that we would use this as the permanent venue for our meetings so, as it was summer, came up with the idea of walking around the block near his home. After a couple of weeks doing this, as I left him and turned to say 'Goodbye', he replied 'Bye' back to me! After a while of this routine I suggested that he come with me to look at a local Learning Centre where they offered computer courses. I thought this environment would be ideal as it was small with very welcoming and friendly staff. William agreed to undertake a BBC Webwise Programme at the learning centre. I sat at the next computer to William working on my own projects and helping him as necessary. William's mother told me that whilst he was at school he had brought books home regularly from their library, so with William's approval we went by taxi to register him at his local library and from then on made a weekly trip to select his books. Initially, I would choose the books, but eventually he took an active part in looking and selecting them for himself. He also became confident enough to go to the counter to bring them back and get the new ones stamped.

Although we had no proper means of communication, we developed our own way around this. William would nod and shake his head, and his range of facial expressions told me a great deal too. I also developed an idea of five 'smiley faces' in a row on a piece of paper. They ranged from downright sad up to really happy. If I wanted to know how strongly he felt for or against something, I pointed to the faces one at a time and he would nod when I was near the face that reflected how he felt. William sailed through the Webwise Programme, so we looked for another course he could study at the Learning Centre.

We had a couple of false starts on courses which turned out to be wrong for William. However, eventually we managed to secure a distance learning CLAIT (computer literacy and information technology) course from a local college using the facilities at the local Learning Centre once more. Again there were difficulties, but William persevered and succeeded in passing the whole course, which was an excellent achievement.

At the end of each term we went out on trips to celebrate the achievements of the past months. The first one was to a local bowling alley in a town a short train ride away. William was very anxious at first, but equally determined that he was going to take an active part in the activity. Eventually, after about 45 minutes of encouragement he bowled the first ball. After this it was plain sailing, even after a group of his peers came to a nearby lane. On the train home he sat by himself and offered the ticket to the attendant himself. We have also visited local museums and always travelled by public transport.

I suggested one week that we could go to a local café to have a drink. William agreed to this but did not want to actually have anything when we got there. After this I asked him if he wanted to go back the next week and he confirmed that he did. The following week he did get a can of Coke and drink it. Every week since then we have done this and William seems to enjoy it.

I was asked to trial a new type of assessment and felt that this would be ideally suited for use with William. He came to my office and I undertook this with him. It was amazing how much information I had actually already gathered from working with him, but it was also very interesting touching on areas that we had not visited before and this gave me a way in to discuss these issues. Through the assessment it was identified that, although he would like to speak to me, our relationship had now become established as a non-speaking one and this was a real barrier to moving forwards. I suggested a couple of ideas about how we could initiate communication to him that I had seen on the selectivemutism.org website but neither seemed to appeal to him. We also identified that William would like to work and eventually live independently. Because of this I put to him the idea that he could go for a psychological work assessment by the Job Centre Plus.

This assessment identified that he needed help and support with his writing skills and spelling. To be effective in the workplace he also needed to have some communication skills. The psychologist also felt a clinical assessment would be beneficial but could not find anyone who dealt with this age group in the area, nor could they find a support group. Without the above, they felt he would not be suitable for placement. I spoke to the psychologist in some detail and she felt that one area that I could look at was his spelling and communication skills. If I played Scrabble with him, getting him to spell out the letters would have a dual purpose.

I managed to find an office which was quiet and local, and initially took William to have a look round to ensure that he felt at ease. He agreed to this and arranged that the following week we would have our first game. When the time came, there was an initial hesitation, but within no time he was putting down the letters and spelling the words out without any problem. As he was so at ease, I asked him also to add up his scores, therefore also improving numeracy. Again, no problem. Therefore I then gave him the target of saying the letters, the score and the whole word – he did it once more.

Shortly after we started our weekly game of Scrabble, he arrived at the office on foot. I asked him how he had got there, ready to go through a list of possibilities which he could nod at accordingly, but he said, 'I walked here'! From what I had read about SM I felt that I should react in a very low-key way to his speech; however, I also felt that it should be acknowledged, so later in the session I brought it into the conversation and told him I was really pleased that he had spoken. He seemed delighted that this achievement was being recognized.

Each week now brought more words into his vocabulary to the point where, when asked, he told me in a couple of complete sentences how he had injured his foot. He has started driving lessons and also regularly walks into town on his own to meet me or on occasions to take back his library books when I am on my annual leave.

I managed to find SMIRA through research one weekend on the internet and contacted them. I was given Alice Sluckin's phone number and spoke to her about the work that I was doing with William. She suggested that I write about the time that William and I have worked together. She also suggested that we purchase the SMIRA video, which we did. It gave me the idea of having some planned responses or 'scripts' for William to use in everyday situations. Most of us accumulate a 'bank' of these responses, but people who have not been speaking in these situations do not. For example: being asked the time or directions from a stranger, or bumping into someone and knocking their shopping to the floor. I wrote out the different scenarios and asked William to tell me what his responses would be. It took a while but he did manage to come up with suitable short answers. We went over them each week until he didn't need to think before he could respond appropriately.

William also started an Adult Education class where he is improving his writing and spelling skills. He attends once a week during the evening and works alongside other adults. This is a wonderful achievement. More recently, he passed his driving theory test and is communicating with his instructor on his driving lessons. He speaks more at home and this has led to much-improved relationships within the family.

Each week I set him small achievable targets (ones that I check are what he wants for himself) and they are usually reached. If they are not, then we look at the reason for not managing something and adapt them or make notes for future reference of what has happened. By doing this we have a wonderful record of everything he has achieved and can easily remind ourselves of the progress he has made. We can see where he was and where he is now, which gives us plenty of scope for celebration.

William has grown much more confident over the past two years. He has always been determined to move on with his life and is constantly amazing me with his progress. We have a mutual respect for each other; he knows that I will never make him do something which he doesn't want to. I give him lots of encouragement and we always take things at his pace. When we first started working together, it seemed as if we had a mountain to climb. We are climbing that mountain one small step at a time, but now we can look down and see how far we have travelled.

It later transpired that, like some other previously SM people, William required further support at transition points in his life.

Talking in the community

Next we describe a group of three children aged 9–12 years old treated by specialist SLT Maggie Johnson.

They were clearly anxious children who had each responded well to individual support in their various primary schools but were unable to generalize their speaking beyond their one-to-one sessions. It was not until their failure to talk at school was tackled directly at a behavioural level that observable progress began, for rather than nurturing or counselling they needed a structured programme to extend their talking circle and actively manage the transition to the next year group.

Similarly, progress made was confined to the school setting and the children's experience of talking outside their structured sessions was limited to immediate family. In order to generalize the progress they were making and continue to challenge their anxiety, they needed parental and professional support to build their confidence in wider settings. For this reason, the SLT ran group sessions in the summer holiday. The summer school comprised nine one-hour sessions of discussion, role play and real-life practice to enable them to extend their ability to talk to unfamiliar people in the community (Johnson and Wintgens 2001 and personal communication).

The importance of our own responses and attitudes when helping SM children is regularly pointed out. One of the tasks of all helpers is to allow the people who are being helped to grow away from the secure base we have provided, so as to experiment with skills and strategies of their own. The more dependent the helped person was in the beginning, the harder this can sometimes be for the helper. Overprotection is no real help.

Once SM children begin to be able to speak outside their easiest circle of contacts, it is helpful to show them how to extend the range of possible people with whom they might risk contact. The slow pace at which this process sometimes proceeds can lead us to think that more protection will be needed than is actually the case. Keeping in mind that independence is the goal, we can provide the children themselves with a method of grading the steps in their own recovery. For example, even after an initial breakthrough, children can sometimes maintain rather rigid boundaries between people and situations they see as 'safe' and those which still frighten them into silence. Help with constructing a detailed ladder of difficulty can be effective in making it possible for them to experiment with communicating with an ever-widening circle of contacts. Once they understand that some steps are easy, while others are quite demanding and can be left until later, they will be less vulnerable to feelings of failure and discouragement.

The Selective Mutism Resource Manual (Johnson and Wintgens 2001) provides just such a ladder (form 6; see Fig. 16.1, page 260 in this book). The detailed instructions make it clear that some tasks are at a similar level of difficulty – for example, speaking where a teacher might overhear you and speaking to an unfamiliar child – while others involve taking quite large steps – for instance, asking a policeman a question. On pages 292–294 of the Johnson and Wintgens manual, there is a detailed description of how the boy 'D' worked with two other children through such a graded progression toward confident speaking in their locality.

Preparing for success in advance was part of the helper's task. Techniques were taught and the children came to trust that extremely small steps would lead to success.

Confirmation that they were ready to progress and that the therapist would be standing by and would prepare some of the people they must speak to provided a degree of safety.

Individuals in the wider community were primed to respond encouragingly and equipped with understanding of the enormity of the task from the children's point of view. Other unobtrusive contributions from the helper were to:

- encourage the children to work as a mutually supportive but slightly competitive group
- equip them with methods of recording progress
- construct, with them, a hierarchy of easy-to-difficult challenges using form 6
- set up intermediate tasks, practice and role play in preparation for the challenges
- involve parents, friends and other contacts as temporary assistants
- provide the participants with a clear understanding of what would constitute success; for instance, some tasks could be skipped on completion of a more difficult item, but each chosen

task had to be completed three times before any attempt was made to tackle anything perceived as more difficult

- secure a desirable final reward for each successful child.

As most formerly SM children find that the key to talking confidently in really unfamiliar settings is to be found in breaking down this huge achievement into a manageable number of smaller steps, the Johnson and Wintgens manual, with its detailed photocopiable lists of games and suggestions, has proved invaluable.

Working as a group became useful to these young people by bolstering their courage and motivating them to persist in the face of difficulty. They provided examples for one another, the bravest taking the lead and appearing to fill the most anxious group member with a determination not to be outdone.

Outcomes

Once a behavioural approach was combined with the necessary practice for generalization, all three students made progress.

'D' achieved all his practice targets and spoke to a new teacher on the first day of transfer to secondary school. He has succeeded at university and enjoys a good social life, despite having remained on the quiet side throughout secondary school.

The 12-year-old continued to view herself as SM at secondary school, but blossomed with a fresh start at college. She is now able to communicate in any setting but recognizes that the years she spent feeling isolated from her peers have taken a toll on her self-esteem.

The youngest girl, though naturally quiet and a little shy, was also brave. With a less entrenched pattern of mutism, she was able to lead the others by example, saying such things as, 'Oh OK, I'll do it.' She made rapid progress and was soon discharged from therapy.

Group treatment appeared to help these students to escape from SM, as they were able to motivate and validate one another, as well as improve one another's understanding and awareness of objectives and techniques.

A final example

Lastly, a brief, but inspiring story from Sue Johnson, a Special Educational Needs Co-ordinator (SENCO).

John (not his real name) started school in September 2002 at the age of four. He hadn't attended a nursery school prior to mainstream school, but had been minded by his grandparents whilst his parents worked. He has a sister who is three years older than him who would, on occasion, speak for him. John refused to speak to any adult at school. He did speak to his peer group, but quickly became silent if an adult was within hearing distance. The class teacher went to see the school SENCO and discussed the problem with her and John's parents, and he was placed on the school's Special Educational Needs register.

There were no particular anxieties at home which could have contributed to the problem, although John's mother had stressed very strongly to her children not to talk to strangers and wondered if she could have over-emphasized this. He was not desperately unhappy at school; he attended every day but didn't like it very much. He did join in all of the activities but refused to speak. Both of John's parents were worried about the situation, fearing that he would fall behind in his school work, especially with his reading.

John's class teacher followed the advice given by SMIRA regarding involvement of parents, use of tape recorders, puppets, etc. John's parents recorded him learning his sounds and reading his book to his mother at home, so that the school would be able to ascertain his educational progress. During this first year at school, John's class teacher encouraged the whole class to respond to the register using non-verbal communication. One day the children would nod their heads, another day they might click their fingers or wink, clap or wave and, as this became part of the classroom routine, John eventually joined in.

By the end of the reception year John had still not spoken to his teacher or any of the other adults within school. He continued to stop talking to his friends as soon as an adult was within hearing distance, although he participated willingly in all activities. John moved into his new class along with his peers and, for the first week or two, the new teacher continued with the non-verbal responses whilst taking the register. The SENCO suggested that the class teacher should try to encourage John to vocalize, but not verbalize at this stage. So, as part of a whole-class activity linked to the literacy hour about 'Old MacDonald's Farm', the children answered the register by quacking like a duck. This was so successful that the children asked if they could continue to do it the following week, but with a different animal. At this stage John still wasn't joining in. However, in the second week, again linked to the literacy hour, the children had to hiss like a snake in answer to the register and John joined in with this voiceless response along with the other children. This was John's fourth term at school and it was the first time any adult had heard him make a sound. The class teacher continued in this way for two or three more weeks. She challenged John gradually to read to a friend whilst she was sitting on a table behind him with her back to him, so that she could hear his reading. Gradually, she moved nearer until eventually she was able to sit next to him.

Within two weeks John was putting up his hand to contribute to the literacy hours. Just before Christmas (i.e. towards the end of his fourth term), he took part in a school assembly, speaking in front of the other children (over 400 of them). John was removed from the Special Needs register at the end of the Spring term, five terms after starting school.

John quickly caught up with his peer group and never regressed. He had lots of friends, with one special friend. He would answer questions when asked, but didn't really volunteer answers. John is now at secondary school, which he enjoys. He works hard, is well behaved, and in a test given in Year 8 (12/13-year-olds) he achieved a reading age of four years ahead of his chronological age. He is happy to speak in front of everyone, excels at spelling and writing, and is more academic than sporty, although he does participate in sports with his friends. One of his favourite subjects is drama, which is one of his options for GCSE (General Certificate of Secondary Education). He hopes to study drama at university with a view to becoming a professional actor.

CHAPTER 10

Successful Combined Home and School Approaches to Selective Mutism

Alice Sluckin and SMIRA Parents

To paraphrase Mark Twin, a habit cannot be tossed out of the window; it must be coaxed down the stairs one step at a time.

Whether one speaks of descending a staircase or climbing a ladder, the key issue in the behavioural approach is gradualness. This chapter gives some inspiring examples of parents and children gaining control of anxiety-related Selective Mutism (SM) by means of 'step at a time' practice.

All children's names have been changed in these examples to provide anonymity.

The story of Peter[1]
TOLD BY ALICE ON THE BASIS OF HIS FATHER'S ACCOUNT

Several of the SM children whose parents have approached SMIRA have had other diagnosed conditions. Peter was such a child.

At birth, he was found to have a cleft lip and palate, a condition that occurs once in 600 to 700 births (Royal College of Speech and

---

1   Not his real name.

Language Therapists 2006; McWilliams, Morris and Shelton 1990; Watson 2001).

This necessitated a repair operation soon after birth, followed by several other admissions to hospital. Cleft palate can interfere with articulation and there is a greatly increased risk of 'glue ear' due to malformation of the Eustacian tubes. At 18 months Peter had grommets inserted into his eardrums, and his response to hearing better was dramatic. He quickly learnt to speak, with a good vocabulary in English and Spanish, his mother's native language.

However, on starting nursery aged three, he did not speak to his teacher or peers, even though he appeared to enjoy being with the other children. He continued not speaking on transfer to primary school. At home he spoke fluently to the family, as well as to visitors. The parents reported no other problems.

As no one at school was able to offer help for Peter, his parents became increasingly concerned for him. By chance, they happened to come across the term 'Selective Mutism' in a Local Authority booklet on special needs, and learnt about our charity SMIRA which was said to help the parents of affected children. The parents contacted us and were given our handouts which explained that SM was, in most cases, likely to be caused by anxiety about speaking at school, and that children could be helped by teachers and parents working together using a step-by-step approach.

Peter's father then suggested to the teacher that they should put into operation a step-by-step programme to help the boy overcome his fear of talking at school. The father said he was willing to join his son's class for three half-hour reading sessions each week and both the teacher and the boy were happy about this plan. Initially, the father saw Peter alone and the boy only managed to whisper in his ear, but after only two weeks he was able to read out loud in a corner of the classroom as long as they were alone. After a while, Peter agreed that one of his classmates could join them, but became silent when this happened. However, after only another two weeks, he began to use a normal voice in this boy's presence. Gradually, more children were introduced, and Peter eventually managed to read and talk in groups of four or five classmates. At this stage an ancillary teacher joined this small group, although she did nothing active at first. After two terms Peter was able to read and speak even when the teacher was leading the group and his father could leave without affecting his confidence and willingness to take part.

Peter's progress in the small group continued steadily, but at a frustratingly slow pace. He still couldn't talk to his peers in the playground or when the whole class was present and he had never spoken to his form teacher. On the plus side, his attitude to school was very positive and he had become an enthusiastic drummer. The breakthrough came when a new and more understanding teacher asked him to perform in class on the drums. This went well, and his enjoyment of the experience seemed to help him to overcome his residual anxiety. The transfer to secondary school caused no further difficulties with communication and he settled happily there. From Sixth Form College, he achieved the advanced qualifications that he needed, and was accepted for the university course of his choosing.

This programme was carried out by a devoted family, with the school's help, over a period of several years. Peter's father also became a member of the SMIRA committee, using his experience to help other parents worried about their children's SM.

The story of Ann[2]
INTRODUCED BY ALICE AND TOLD BY HER MOTHER WHO HELPED BY NOT GIVING IN TO ANXIETY

The next example involves a quite different type of person who behaved from an early age like a typical SM child. With regard to causation, she was probably genetically predisposed to being excessively anxious. She may have been 'behaviourally inhibited to the unfamiliar', a condition present in 10–15 per cent of newborns (Kagan and Snidman 2004). These children have a lower physiological threshold of reactivity with regard to fearfulness, especially in new situations, which explains their behaviour. It is thought that a percentage of SM children belong to this group.

Having already brought up a child, Ann's mother was able to resist the trap of overprotecting her daughter. Instead, she lovingly and gently encouraged gradual exposure to mildly anxiety-

---

2   Not her real name.

provoking situations. The expectation she conveyed to Ann was that she would gain the confidence to succeed in time, which she did.

Like Peter, Ann was brought up in a loving, child-centred home. With this help and that of her school she overcame, step-by-step, her fear of unfamiliar people and situations.

Here is Ann's story, as told by her mother.

We have now been free of SM for over a year. People used to tell me that once the child started speaking, it was amazing how quickly things progressed. I never believed them, until I saw it for myself. I once heard Maggie Johnson speaking and she said for most children with SM, one day it becomes such a dim and distant memory that the ex-sufferer can hardly believe it ever happened in the first place. I was even less inclined to believe that, but I think if I were to tell my daughter what it was like for her three years, two years or even 18 months ago, she would think I was making it up.

I would like to stress that in my experience, with lots of hard work, time and dedication from the child and their family, you can get over it, completely.

We have a happy, stable family with a Mum and a Dad and three children; three chickens, a cat and a rabbit. My middle child, my only daughter, is the child who suffered from SM. She is nearly eight years old as I write this. I feel that my daughter Ann was born with SM, but it wasn't until she was around three years old that I realized it was more than just 'her personality'. (I didn't have a diagnosis – a staff member at play-school said she thought it was SM and I Googled it. It was like reading a description of my daughter!) We worked intensely, aiding recovery from when she was around three years old, and the recovery process began with significant steps in the spring of 2012 when she was six years old. Until that point nothing that I tried ever worked at all, but I kept on trying, hoping that one day it would. And sure enough, there came a point when she was ready.

My daughter was always aware that she had SM, that other children had it and that it would get better. I always stressed that the older you got, the better you got at everything, talking included. I told her that there was no rush and that everyone would be patient, but that one day she would need to tackle her fear. I encouraged and pushed and gave her opportunity wherever I could. I never ever used SM as an excuse for anything. We would find a way around everything so that Ann didn't ever miss out on something because of the SM.

Until 2012, Ann had only ever spoken to 11 adults and six children in her whole life. Up until then she was unable to speak to aunties, uncles or any other family members, family friends, neighbours, shop assistants, other mums, any staff at school – the list is endless. She was always able to speak to my husband and me and to her two brothers, and eventually she was able to speak to three close friends she made at play-school after many, many play dates, but only out of earshot and sight of school staff!

Whilst Ann was suffering from SM she was able, once comfortable with a person, to communicate non-verbally with nods and shakes of the head and pointing but could not attempt any more complex forms of non-verbal communication. For instance, she was not able to perform the actions to songs, or wave hello/goodbye to people. At home Ann always was, and still is, extremely chatty, happy, funny, energetic and rather bossy! She is loud and talks excessively. All through the lifetime of her condition, when we went out as a family to places where she felt she was anonymous, she would be very loud and very much herself, often the loudest child in the café/supermarket/on the beach. I think she perhaps felt safe in the knowledge that she would never see these people again.

I can remember attending SMIRA events when Ann was three years old, then four, then five and being in the same position every year with very little, if any, progress made each year.

I can remember when Ann was five years old and we'd been attempting to tackle it for over two years. At one of the annual SMIRA meetings I was saying that we were no further forward, but I recall that a man who was attending who had an older child recovering from SM said that you may not see the progress now, but perhaps when she is older, that's when it will all pay off. He could not have been more right! So even if you see no results of your efforts, from experience I believe that all the effort is likely to be small building blocks leading very slowly to recovery.

We did not get any professional help – I would advise that you do not let this worry you too much! Become your own professional. Read up, buy literature and take the lead. Do not wait around for appointments with anyone! Get started, as recovery takes so long there is no time to waste. Over the last four years I obviously did a lot of research; I contacted SMIRA, I went to SMIRA events and also, as I live in Leicestershire, I joined the SMIRA committee. I approached my daughter's school before she had even started there, and I set in motion the things I thought would help Ann. In the 16 weeks prior to her starting school, we visited the classroom once a week for 20 minutes after school where I, my daughter and her brothers (and eventually just I and my daughter and finally just my daughter and the TA) played alongside the teaching assistant in the classroom. I was always very aware when dealing with the school that Ann was one of over 400 children in the school; I did not expect any special treatment or even too much extra time. I appreciated how busy everyone was. I put in all the work.

I drafted the IEPs (Individual Education Plans), I made the suggestions, I drafted and went in to lead the 'sliding-in' programme. When I made suggestions that they couldn't accommodate, I simply put forward a suggestion that involved less of their time.

The key points from my experience would be firstly and perhaps most importantly that progress is very slow, and steps of progress taken are so small you can barely see them. I was only ever able to measure that there had been any progress of any kind by looking on an annual basis, when I could say, for example, that this year she can wave hello and last year she was unable to. I would say to always bear this in mind. Just because you have been trying a strategy and it hasn't worked yet doesn't mean to say that it is not going to work or be of some benefit in the future. Even tiny, insignificant steps are still steps.

Second (and I think it is equally as key), keep at the forefront of your mind that SM should be temporary. Try not to define your child by it or use it as a reason for your child not to do something – there are ways around everything! I treated all three of my children the same: they all learned to ride their bikes, they all had swimming lessons, they all bought their own chocolate bar in the shop – the only difference was that Ann did it silently! I have never made allowances or exceptions because of Ann's SM. This helped to build my daughter's confidence and this way she always knew I had confidence in her. She always felt she could do anything she wanted to do. Why on earth not?

I believe that another important part of recovery is to get the child to take responsibility themselves. Nobody wants to do something that cripples them with fear; it's much easier to just avoid it altogether. But I think it needs to be made clear that you cannot live your life this way. I have heard SM parents supporting their child's difference, saying everyone is different and that is fine. But a life not speaking to anyone – that was not going to be fine for my daughter. I was not prepared to celebrate this difference!

From the beginning, Ann was aware that she had SM. I also made it clear that it was a temporary thing, that others had it, that everyone was scared of something and that eventually that something became less scary. When she was around six years old and I felt she was mature enough, I made it clear that no one would put pressure on her and that she could do it in her own time but she would HAVE to overcome her fears, there was no choice in this matter. I began to introduce more steps and strategies which took her on her journey very, very slowly. I never stopped gently pushing and challenging her and getting the teachers to do the same.

From the age of five years until she was seven years she took a herbal remedy that claimed to relieve anxiety and shyness in children. We called them her 'brave' tablets and said they would eventually make her feel more brave about talking. Within four weeks of taking them she made her first 'sound' (a nonsense sound during a phonics lesson) at school so I definitely feel that they had an impact, whether actual or placebo. Prior to taking them she could not even make a sound at school, not a cough or an animal noise.

Another key thing for us was that I spent a long period of time trying to bribe or offer rewards for things – and it simply did not work, she could not be bribed. But then we reached a point in the journey where she began to seem open to the offer of an incentive for very small steps that I was trying to encourage her to do – for example, hand a note to a teacher, take in a Dictaphone message.

She collected 'Hello Kitty' stickers in an album and they were bought as a reward each time she did a very small step. A significant and more long-term incentive was that she wanted her ears pierced and I told her that I would have liked her to be around nine years old. But then I added that if she worked really hard at overcoming her fears, at the end of the school year when she had made enough progress that she could do everything in school that she needed to speaking-wise, she could have them done, however old she was. I said that there was no rush. She had them pierced one year later at the age of six and a half!

For us, small, painfully slow steps were the key. We didn't rush any of the steps and we didn't move on until she was totally comfortable with the step we were tackling. But I did make sure that I was constantly gently pushing and challenging her. The process, for me, was exhausting and constant. I never ever stopped thinking or planning – even through the night!

Ann did not speak or make a sound for all her play-school years and the entire first year of her primary school life. Now, aged almost eight years, she will respond with speech to anyone. And that's anyone in the school or anyone outside of the school. Whilst her answers may not be long, whilst she still may appear like a quiet, shy girl when she asks a question (she is not!), she can do it. She even takes on speaking parts in school plays! Who would have thought it was ever possible?

In my experience, small steps that seem to lead to nowhere are the way forward. Here are some of the examples of small steps that we practised in school to get Ann able to speak to staff in the school:

1. In 2012 (Ann's second year at school), pass notes to the two teaching staff in her class. She was not required to speak, merely to hand over the note to a staff member she was familiar with. Even this was a challenge at first.

2. Once she was comfortable with the physical passing of notes, we told her she must read the note out to the receiving teacher and the teacher ensured that she was looking away from Ann (back turned) as she read. Reading a script usually holds less pressure as it is the uncertainty of what to say which causes us all most concern. She did this for a number of weeks. It wasn't easy, and took quite a few attempts, with a few barely audible messages passed!

3. We then moved on to reading the note out to the teacher with the teacher facing Ann directly. This was a big challenge and was practised for a number of weeks.

4. Then we asked Ann to memorize the note and re-tell it to the teacher, keeping the note in her hand.

5. We then asked Ann to put the note down on a desk before re-telling the contents of it to the teacher. This step once again lasted a number of weeks.

6. Then the teaching staff got her to pass the message without a written note. The first time this was requested of her, I'm told, she looked a little bewildered, but the teacher stood firm and asked her to quickly do it. She did.

    They did this for weeks until Ann was totally comfortable with passing on verbal messages between her own teacher and her own teaching assistant. From this point there seemed to be an easy transition from being able to repeat something the teacher had asked her to say to her being able to just say something that she wanted to say when the teacher asked her a question.

7. Then they moved the scenario out of Ann's classroom and the steps were carried out around the school to the Head, to other teachers and to the office staff. Notes were passed; then read; then messages repeated. We found that as she had already completed the process in her own classroom, she was able to repeat the steps very quickly outside of the classroom. Generalizing to the rest of the school took just a couple of weeks.

For Ann, this process was in small enough steps that she was then eventually able to function very well around the school. I did a similar process at home, encouraging her to do more interaction in shops, cafés and with family members.

Once this process started (around March 2012), it was incredible how quickly her new-found skills transferred into other situations and the boundaries of what she was able to do blurred; she was soon answering questions at school and offering information to her teachers. We had no part in this; she simply did it herself.

In June 2012 she asked if I thought she had conquered her fears enough to have her ears pierced. She was still unable to answer the register at this point. I told her that she would need to answer the register too before she could have them done. I can still remember the look of horror on her face, but I knew it was important that I pushed her. One week later she pushed herself enough to do it; she was very determined!

As I have already said, I know that now she has trouble remembering how it used to be. We don't talk about it at all anymore – I made a decision not to refer to it after the ear piercing, so that she was able to move on and re-create herself. She had no trouble transferring years at school last year or this (into the juniors – I haven't even been in to see her new teacher!), and last month Ofsted (school inspectors) visited her school and they randomly chose her to read and then answer questions about the story she had read to them. I'm told she did it like a professional!

Animals helping children to talk at school and with unfamiliar people

Touching and relating to undemanding animals has long been thought to soothe disturbed emotions. Interestingly, the University of Leicester was recently seen to provide a small 'petting zoo' during the examination period, having been told that students could derive benefit from just this type of interaction. Over the years, we have heard of several SM children appearing to be given confidence by relating to pets who could not possibly put them under any pressure. A selection of such stories is included here.

Becky (not her real name) was seven years old and lived with loving parents who were members of SMIRA. She had been diagnosed as having SM at the age of three as she did not speak at nursery and had hardly improved when starting primary school. The parents then read that children with SM responded well to pets. Though not having had a pet before, they decided to add a dog to their small family and Becky was delighted. Once they had acquired Bobby, the news spread in the neighbourhood and children came to the door to make Bobby's acquaintance. This led to Becky acquiring new friends and she began to speak to them. The next high point was Becky being asked by the teacher to give a talk about Bobby to the class. She was able to speak clearly and with confidence. This was a real breakthrough for her and from then on she continued to make steady progress.

The parents were greatly relieved and shared their joy with SMIRA.

Another child diagnosed with SM found the confidence to speak after his SENCO recommended that he should attend therapeutic donkey-riding as well as seeing an SLT. It was hoped that, by learning how to give instructions to the animal, the boy would lose his fear of talking. As predicted, he started to whisper 'Stop' and 'Start' and was able to get louder, shouting instructions at times. Within a year, he was speaking to children in the playground and answered his teachers when they asked questions.

This family appears to have been helped by speech and language therapy and the Elizabeth Swendsen Trust for Children and Donkeys which has riding therapy centres in Birmingham, Ivybridge, Manchester, Sidmouth and Leeds.

Another family who are members of SMIRA includes a son with SM and Asperger Syndrome who had begun to talk after being seen by an SLT who started him on a programme derived from the Johnson and Wintgens (2001) manual. He responded well to this and began to talk at school.

Unfortunately, he had been discharged by the SLT department, although like many SM children, he was apt to relapse into silence at every transition point in his school life – for example, on joining a new class or meeting a new teacher.

The situation was saved when the family acquired a kitten. Very soon, boy and cat became close friends as she was spending most of her time in his room. The boy was heard speaking to his pet and this was probably what eventually led to his becoming able to express some of his feelings and starting to talk again at school with his peers and with the teacher.

The thorough preparation which had been undertaken previously via the Breaking Down the Barriers programme will also have played a part.

The mother has written a book about the way her son has managed to overcome SM with the help of their pet. In a prologue, she describes the boy giving a most competent talk at school about 'Jessi-Cat'. The book is *The Cat that Unlocked a Boy's Heart: Jessi-Cat* by Jayne Dillon with Alison Malony (2013).

The Story of Holly[3]
INTRODUCED BY ALICE AND
CONTINUED BY THE FAMILY

The final example tells the story of a family who had to cope for years, as many families do, without recognition of SM and even with feelings of blame and criticism. Eventually, they heard about the step-by-step approach through SMIRA, and came across an enlightened teacher with 20 years' experience who worked with the child with great success. The account shows what a difference an excellent school can make to an SM child and her worried family.

Like many SM children who fully recover, Holly is anxious to tell her story, hoping that it will benefit other children. Here is her story, as told by her parents, and continued by Holly herself.

When Holly was at nursery, it was brought to our attention that she didn't speak to the teachers, but we didn't worry about it. When she spoke to her friends, but not to teachers, at primary school, we got no support from the school; in fact, they made us feel it was our fault. This went on for two years and ended with a blazing row with the Head. Because of this, we moved Holly to a small village school where she was much happier, but she still didn't speak. By Year 4 we moved her again to fit in with her sister's transfer to secondary school and the new staff were much more supportive. Holly joined one of the school clubs and the teacher who ran it told us about SMIRA.

I phoned Lindsay Whittington at SMIRA, who was great. We got the DVD *Silent Children* and all the information. When Holly started Year 6, her teacher was brilliant. She took the DVD home, cried, and was ready to work with us. She gave up time after school and we did the 'sliding-in' method. By the end of the first week, Holly was in the classroom on her own reading to this teacher. Their co-operation went on for months; they read, played games and went round the school meeting the rest of the staff, who built up our daughter's confidence by chatting with her.

When the time came to change classes, both teacher and pupil were crying and hugging each other because they knew that a real difference had been made.

---

3   Not her real name.

Holly is now 12 and nearly ready to leave Year 7. The teacher in her new class was also lovely and worked with us from the start. She arranged to meet us the day before term started in an empty school. Holly has done really well. She has sung with the choir in a variety of venues, enjoys drama and has given a ten-minute presentation at school about one of her interests, baking.

We want children and families where SM is a problem to know that, with the right approach, there is light at the end of the tunnel. Holly herself has kindly written this letter:

Dear SMIRA,

I am very proud of myself since I started Year 6 because last year was the very first time I had spoken to a teacher, or even near one. I spoke only quietly, but it was still such a big step for me that I cried with happiness.

Then I stayed after school a few nights each week to play games with my teacher. One night, I decided I was confident enough to talk to the Head Teacher. I walked to her office with Mrs Walker, and when I spoke to her she was so happy. I realized then what a long way I had come and decided I could speak to other teachers too, so I did.

Then I decided that I wasn't going to let anything stop me joining the children's choir because I love singing. The teacher who runs the choir seemed scary at first and I didn't want to sing to her on my own, but after about a month I thought 'I can do this', so I sang in front of her. It was quite quiet, but I still did it and that's what counted for me and since I started this letter I have moved up to the girls' choir.

When the big day came to leave primary school, I was sad to leave my kind teacher and all the other staff I had got to know. I was worried that I was going to get scared in the bigger school and not be confident enough to ask someone where to go. Luckily, I found my way around after about two weeks. The important thing about starting secondary school is that I have started afresh and talked to the teachers the first time I met them and never looked back.

I'm having a lot more fun at school now and I've made tons of new friends. It's like opening up a whole new world. I'm a lot happier since I started talking to the teachers at school.

MY ACHIEVEMENTS

- Now I can go up to the corner shop by myself and buy a newspaper.

- The other day I went up and ASKED for a mobile phone top-up.

- I have joined the choir, talked at school, sung by myself, talked to shop owners.

- I've been to the supermarket by myself.

- In drama (my favourite subject) I've taken the role of the narrator.

- With the choir, I've performed in the opera house.

- At school, I've spoken in front of the whole class.

- I'm going to be one of the people showing the new children around the school.

So, I really want to help other children like me and tell them that there's nothing to be scared of. I'm sure teachers will be happy when you talk to them and there are people who will help you and be happy to do so.

I want you to understand that there's a pot of gold at the end of the rainbow. I know it's hard, but you can do it.

Well, that's my story and I hope it helps other children and families.

Thank you for all the help and support you've given me. From Holly

CHAPTER 11

Effective Care Pathways for Selective Mutism

Maggie Johnson, Miriam Jemmett and Charlotte Firth

Introduction

'Care pathways' represent a turning point in ensuring quality and equity of healthcare. By describing how local services will provide for a particular condition, care pathways standardize local practice and inform individuals of the support they can expect to receive.

In 2008, an international consensus-based care pathway of good practice for Selective Mutism (SM) was developed by Keen, Fonseca and Wintgens. The aim was to agree and validate key principles underlying the assessment and management of SM through a consensus process involving international experts, in order to create a local care pathway.

Thirteen recognized experts from North America, Europe and Australia participated in the process and agreement was reached on 11 key principles for an SM care pathway.

The aim of this chapter is to explore how these principles have been applied in the development of SM care pathways in the UK and provide a framework for establishing effective local provision.

As practising speech and language therapists (SLTs) from different NHS Trusts in the North and South of England, the authors have all been involved in developing more robust provision for children with SM. Aware that we were not alone, we invited professionals to share their local care pathways via the Royal College of Speech and Language Therapists (RCSLT) and contacts with education services who had requested training in SM. We have been greatly encouraged by the various contributions that have been made to this chapter, but are aware that SM remains relatively poorly understood. These children still 'fall through the gaps' in terms of service provision, with much debate about professional remit and ownership of the condition. We therefore conclude with a flow diagram, which we recommend as a starting point for teams wishing to develop their own care pathway.

Setting the scene

Effective care planning can only be achieved after general awareness-raising about the existence of SM and long-term implications if left untreated. In the last eight years alone there have been a number of moves in the UK which have significantly raised the profile of SM on a national basis. All have been achieved by a few individuals campaigning together as clinical experts and SMIRA representatives:

1. The RCSLT followed the American Speech–Language–Hearing Association's lead and included SM within the professional remit of SLTs (RCSLT 2006).

2. SM was added to the NHS Choices A–Z of conditions, giving online access to information and appropriate management of the condition, including the need for education and health services to work in collaboration with families.

3. The National Institute for Health and Care Excellence guidelines for the treatment of social anxiety disorder included reference to SM, alerting health practitioners to the need to consider SM as an alternative or additional diagnosis.

4. The Communication Trust included SM in the range of speech, language and communication needs that would benefit from their support in securing appropriate management and legislation.

The impact of local awareness-raising initiatives and campaigns for service provision has been greatly enhanced with this national backing.

The international consensus – core recommendations

For the purposes of this chapter we have summarized Keen *et al.'s* (2008) 11 key principles under five broader headings, each of which will be discussed with specific examples of good practice:

- A multi-modal and multi-agency approach to assessment and intervention with local agreement on the first point of contact for those seeking advice and support.

- Provision of training to educate all involved in identifying and supporting children with SM.

- Access to an individualized intervention programme as soon as SM is identified, with an emphasis on parental involvement in real-life settings.

- Progress determined by improved social functioning.

- Access to a dedicated support group or organization such as the Selective Mutism Information & Research Association (SMIRA).

A multi-modal approach to assessment and intervention
International consensus recommendations (Keen *et al.* 2008):

Each area should agree a specific service or group of professionals who are the first point of contact to advise educational settings and confirm that a child has SM.

Children with SM must receive a thorough assessment, which considers the possibility of co-existing difficulties such as developmental delay and other communication difficulties. Full consideration must be given to all possible relevant factors such as having English as an additional language and any emotional or behavioural difficulties. If there are found to be other difficulties alongside the SM, additional intervention must be provided as appropriate, as well as specific intervention for the SM.

If a child does not make the expected progress despite provision of an appropriate programme for their SM, it will be important to consider the possibility of co-existing difficulties or factors that may be having an impact. If progress is felt to be hampered by severe levels of anxiety, for example, a therapeutic trial of medication (i.e. SSRIs) may be appropriate. Any such additional intervention should be provided in addition to a behavioural programme and should not replace it.

The first step towards such a multi-modal approach is to create a multi-agency team committed to joined-up thinking about the needs of SM children, with an awareness of each other's roles and remit. At the heart of SM is a communication difficulty – difficulty talking to or in front of certain people as a result of learned anxiety – but there are often additional considerations such as high sensitivity, communication disorders, co-ordination difficulties, second-language learning and other anxieties. Good practice therefore starts with informal multi-agency discussion, leading to more formal meetings to agree a model based on local networks, resources and expertise, followed by workshops and information days to develop information leaflets, raise awareness and share agreed policy, including specific referral criteria for each agency involved.

The majority of care pathways we have seen direct initial referrals towards SLTs (see example in Figure 11.1) but Educational Psychologists (EPs) or Child and Adolescent Mental Health Services (CAMHS) take the lead in other areas of the UK. Some SLTs only accept referrals when co-morbid speech, language or communication difficulties are suspected (see example in Figure 11.2).

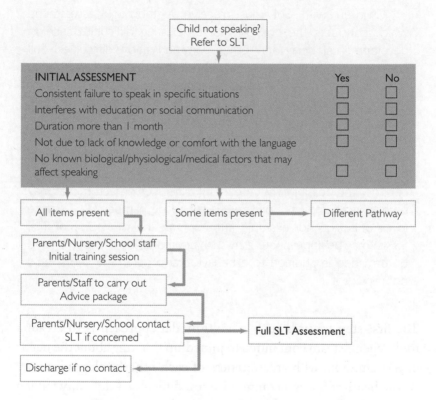

Figure 11.1 East Sussex care pathway: initial
identification and referral route

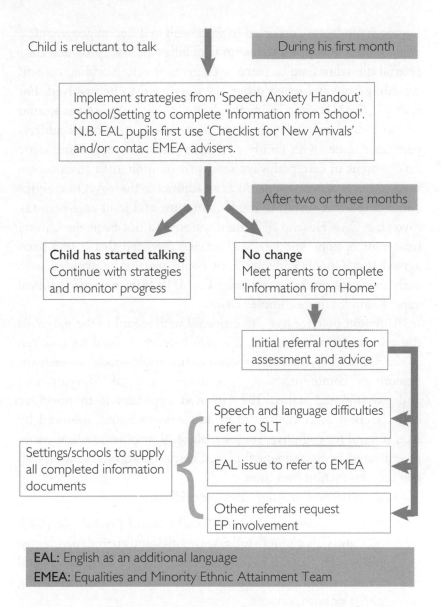

Child is reluctant to talk

During his first month

Implement strategies from 'Speech Anxiety Handout'.
School/Setting to complete 'Information from School'.
N.B. EAL pupils first use 'Checklist for New Arrivals'
and/or contac EMEA advisers.

After two or three months

Child has started talking
Continue with strategies
and monitor progress

No change
Meet parents to complete
'Information from Home'

Initial referral routes for
assessment and advice

Speech and language difficulties
refer to SLT

Settings/schools to supply
all completed information
documents

EAL issue to refer to EMEA

Other referrals request
EP involvement

EAL: English as an additional language
EMEA: Equalities and Minority Ethnic Attainment Team

Figure 11.2 Suffolk care pathway: initial intervention and referral routes

Different models are reported to work well in different geographical areas. It does not appear to matter who takes the lead, provided clear referral guidelines are in place with prompt action and agreement regarding how and when other agencies need to be involved. For example, CAMHS may be involved when there are questions around co-morbidity with other mental health difficulties or to address particular issues with family dynamics and parenting. Psychiatric involvement in care pathways seems to be limited to cases where medication is being considered as an adjunct to therapy. One service commented that since the implementation of a joint care pathway involving CAMHS and SLT, medication had not been the chosen treatment option. Another SLT service reported that it had been agreed that CAMHS involvement could usually be avoided with early intervention, but their local CAMHS team provided clinical supervision for more complex cases.

Different practice has also emerged with regard to the nature of the assessment process itself. It would be very unusual for children in the UK to automatically receive a full multi-modal assessment exploring communication, cognition, general development and psychosocial status. The favoured approach is to prioritize consideration of communication and anxiety issues, followed by later referral for cognitive, sensory, physical or other medical issues as indicated by assessment findings, response to intervention and general observation over time.

Four initial assessment routes are evident:

- *Joint assessment involving SLT and Clinical Psychologist (CP).* SLT and CP conduct a full assessment jointly or independently, followed by liaison to formulate a diagnosis, consider referral to other agencies and agree a management plan involving either or both services.

- *Child-focused assessment with a designated service.* SLT, EP, CP or Minority Ethnic Achievement Service assesses the child within the context of their own specialism. Observations and parental interview will ascertain the need for onward referral to other agencies for additional assessment.

- *Parent-focused assessment with a designated service.* As above but the initial focus is on establishing a diagnosis of SM via comprehensive interviews with parents and other key personnel (e.g. class teacher) rather than conducting a face-to-face assessment with the child. Screening questions are asked to decide if full assessment is indicated for any aspect of the child's development, but the onus is on implementing appropriate intervention as soon as possible without burdening the child with the additional anxiety of meeting a stranger. Should further assessment prove necessary it may be deferred, as it is recognized that findings are unreliable when children are anxious.

- *Unofficial diagnosis and management, with the option of assessment.* This approach is only recommended in tandem with a rolling universal training programme (see next section). Participants are provided with guidelines for diagnosis and intervention, with clear criteria for requesting specialist assessment and support. This non-invasive approach allows children to work with the people they see on a day-to-day basis in familiar environments and ensures that specialist time is reserved for more complex cases.

These approaches share the pragmatic view that as long as all aspects of a multi-modal assessment are considered, it is not necessary to conduct a full multi-modal assessment routinely. The approaches differ in scope and timing, each balancing the risk of overlooking relevant contributory factors against the risk of delaying intervention. All approaches have their merits, but we observe that, as general awareness in the community increases, the need to officially diagnose SM decreases.

Provision of training

International consensus recommendations (Keen *et al.* 2008):

> As early identification is key in the successful management of SM, and as it is usually within the pre-school or school setting where the mutism manifests itself, it is important that pre-school and school staff receive training to develop their awareness of how to recognize SM. Awareness-raising training should also present accurate information about what does and doesn't cause SM, and how it should be managed within the educational setting. As it will often be pre-school or school staff who raise the issue with a child's parents, it is important that they know how to do this with confidence and sensitivity.
>
> There is also a need for ongoing training and professional development amongst the professionals who will be involved in supporting these pre-school and school staff.

We have received many examples of services engaged in awareness-raising amongst pre-schools, schools and parents. Activities include the distribution of information leaflets to support parents and staff in the early identification and management of SM, and universal training to which all local schools and pre-schools are invited, regardless of whether or not these settings have children with SM on roll. Services have commented that it is through attending these training days that staff realize they do know children with SM or at risk of developing it. This is a very positive impact of training, which will ultimately lead to prevention, as reluctance to speak will not be maintained through inappropriate emphasis on talking (Cline and Baldwin 2004).

Services are also delivering targeted training 3–4 times a year as part of their care pathway, inviting staff and parents of identified children with SM. Some services do not accept referrals for specific casework until interested parties have attended an initial training session and implemented appropriate strategies. This demonstrates to parents and staff that they are integral to helping their child move forward and minimizes waiting time for accessing specialist advice.

Some services combine half- and full-day training sessions, with parents and staff of pre-school children attending only the morning session which focuses on awareness-raising and general environmental modifications. When these attendees leave before the session on formal small-steps interventions, it acts as a powerful reminder that SM can be successfully treated without the need for formal programmes, if identified and supported early enough. In an audit of SM cases carried out in 2013 by East Kent Hospitals University NHS Foundation Trust (EKHUFT) SLT service, 13 out of 15 children referred as pre-schoolers had overcome their difficulties by their sixth birthday with the support of this training.

Services also recognize the need for training and ongoing clinical supervision amongst the professionals who are taking the 'expert' roles for SM – for example, SLTs or psychologists. The Universal SLT service within Kent Community Health NHS Trust (KCHT) conducted a survey amongst its staff in 2013 which revealed a direct correlation between training and confidence levels amongst the therapists. One training tool that has proved to be particularly useful in building confidence amongst professionals is the use of video to demonstrate specific techniques.

Within the UK there is now a framework for SM training for professionals, with University College London hosting a two-day programme each year within the Division of Psychology and Language Sciences. This training is mainly attended by SLTs and psychologists, who cascade the information down to their teams.

In some areas of the UK, professionals have set up local interest groups to provide peer supervision and continuing professional development. One example of this is a SLT-led Kent-wide interest group, which has also been attended by professionals from specialist teaching services, CAMHS and child health. It should not be forgotten that, although each agency's primary focus will be on supporting children and families, practitioners also need support to share the responsibility of case-management in an area which can be intellectually and emotionally draining for all concerned.

Access to individualized intervention programmes in real-life settings

International consensus recommendations (Keen *et al.* 2008):

SM needs to be treated as soon as it is identified in order to minimize anxiety for the child, their family and their teachers. Early intervention is more likely to be effective and will reduce the need for more lengthy and complex interventions with older children. Treatment strategies need to be implemented in the day-to-day settings where SM occurs, for example in the child's home, pre-school or school setting, and monitored via frequent planning meetings. Mutism may be perpetuated by the behaviours and responses of family and teachers and generates negative feelings in the adults involved; parents and school staff should therefore be involved in the intervention process, supported by specialist clinicians or advisors.

Although far from standard practice, many services across the UK are now providing comprehensive packages of care for children with SM and their families.

Common themes which emerge are:

- Confidence in the evidence-based behavioural principles embraced by *The Selective Mutism Resource Manual* (Johnson and Wintgens 2001).

  This practical guide helps parents and professionals reduce children's anxiety and gradually increase their comfort with talking. The KCHT survey which involved 48 SLTs treating a total of 123 children with SM indicated that these techniques were 91 per cent successful in extending the child's talking circle, increasing to 96.5 per cent successful if the SLT had attended a full training day. When the techniques were not successful, it was noted that the manual guidance had not been followed (e.g. intervention sessions were inconsistent or infrequent) or that the situation was complicated by the long-standing nature of the SM and the mental health status of the student or parent.

- A focus on early intervention and prevention.

  Services are aware that by dispelling the myth that it is safe to wait for young children to 'outgrow' SM, the need for more costly or extended intervention at a later date will be reduced. Various initiatives are in place to provide early years settings with appropriate management techniques to support all quiet children as soon as reluctance to speak is noted (see Johnson and Jones 2012). Posters in general practitioner (GP) and health centre waiting rooms, information leaflets on Trust websites and training sessions for early years workers are used to encourage early referral.

- An emphasis on environmental adaptation as a precursor and backdrop to individual treatment programmes.

  It is recognized that treatment programmes will be ineffective while the child experiences general anxiety or specific anxiety about talking. It is therefore essential to aim for safe, loving and stable home and school environments, and look specifically at adult behaviour that may be maintaining fear or avoidance of talking. 'Creating the right environment' is a powerful but low-key intervention which usually effects an immediate reduction in anxiety levels, enabling the child to benefit fully from individual rapport-building or treatment sessions (see example in Figure 11.3). Here the focus of intervention is to help families and early years staff modify their own interaction with the child, so that the child feels under no pressure to communicate but experiences many positive and enjoyable associations with communication. Avoidance is not an option! Rather, parents and staff facilitate participation by making activities more manageable for the child and responding positively to non-verbal communication, until the child feels more comfortable about talking. This is accompanied by desensitization to speaking in public using voice-activated toys and recording devices, for example, and by setting up situations where the child can talk to their parents or friends without fear of being directly questioned by other people present.

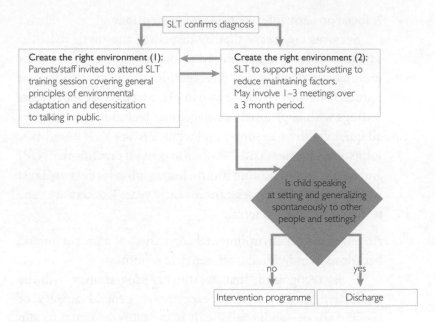

Figure 11.3 Extract from EKHUFT care pathway

- Recognition that specialists are usually best placed to advise on the planning and delivery of intervention programmes, rather than working directly with the child.

   Taking a consultative rather than hands-on role reflects expert opinion that children with SM will only overcome their fear of talking if they gradually face the fear in the social situations where the fear occurs. It is not uncommon to find that children with SM are able to talk to outside professionals in a clinic setting, enabled by the comforting presence of their parent, the removal of an audience, and the clinician's skill in reducing anxiety by only gradually increasing the communication expectations. Continuing to work with a clinician in a clinic setting has very limited value for the child with SM, as it adds only one new person to their talking circle – a person who plays no part in their day-to-day life.

   Eliciting speech with one individual is only the start of the process. Children need support to generalize to a range of people, activities and settings and to use their speech at a functional level to meet their needs. Only adults who see the child on a day-to-day basis are in a good position to facilitate this generalization process; the same adults who are well placed to build rapport, secure the child's trust and be the first person the child talks to in the school setting. Furthermore, adults who are already in frequent contact with the child can provide support over a protracted period of time on a 'little but often' basis which is far more effective than lengthy or infrequent individual sessions (Johnson and Wintgens 2001). They have greater flexibility than outside professionals when it comes to managing the practicalities of delivering a school-based programme, and by taking on the role of key-worker they free the child from the potential stress of engaging with a stranger in an unfamiliar environment. Such commitment to children with SM would not be possible without goodwill, training and ongoing specialist support, but we can be proud that in the UK the resource for this form of service delivery is generally found by schools following the SEN Code of Practice.

However, it can be advantageous for outside professionals to invest time in developing a relationship with the child and eliciting speech by 'sliding-in' as the child talks to a conversational partner (usually the parent). They can provide the family with a model to imitate when 'sliding-in' a friend or family member that the child does not talk to. Using first-hand knowledge of the child's anxiety and comfort triggers, they can repeat the 'sliding-in' process with a school-based member of staff who will take over as key-worker for the generalization phase. Very importantly, they will gain true understanding of the skills and emotional control that are required to be an effective key-worker, improving their effectiveness and confidence as a consultant and support for school-based staff in the future.

Regular support to maintain momentum and quickly address any issues that arise is essential. This is best achieved through multi-agency review meetings and individual e-mail or telephone contact, as demonstrated in Figure 11.4. Review meetings are deemed most effective if embedded in existing educational policy for multi-agency liaison and individual target-setting.

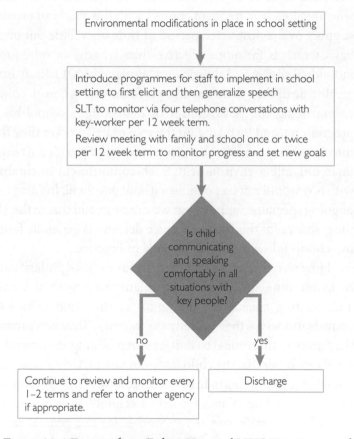

Figure 11.4 Extract from Ealing Hospital NHS Trust care pathway

• Recognition that SM is rarely restricted to the school setting.

Much of the available literature around SM focuses on school as the main setting where children do not speak, and indeed the child's school is the favoured setting in UK care pathways for regular review meetings. However, the information leaflets developed as part of each care pathway emphasize that intervention should also extend to home and community settings. Parents may be advised to invite classmates home, for example, or to facilitate natural talking in public by retreating slightly from onlookers rather than offering a willing ear for whispered communications. They may need examples of how to be positive – for example, 'He'll be able to talk if you make comments rather than asking questions and let him join in his own time' or 'She does it a different way' – rather than speaking negatively in front of their children – for example, 'He won't talk' or 'She can't do that.'

Best practice involves reaching agreement on targets and strategies for both home and school at each review meeting, particularly as our own clinical experience indicates that getting 'stuck' in one setting impinges on progress in other settings. A meeting or phone conversation between parents and their designated contact before the review meeting may well be valued and productive. One care pathway includes a termly group meeting for parents, mediated by a specialist SLT. The success of this is put down to the inspiration and emotional support provided by the participants, rather than the resident 'expert'. The focus is the child's inclusion in family life and the local community; popular themes include: 'letting go' and facilitating independence; helping children manage anxiety rather than eliminating it through avoidance; and the transition to secondary school.

Older children tend to benefit from a mentor rather than parent to support them in achieving targets in their local community – these should be planned according to the student's personal goals and priorities, be this following a chosen interest or career, using the telephone, shopping or travelling independently, or making friends. This is an area which does not seem to be well developed in current care pathways but we know of individual cases where this mentor role has been taken on by school-based support staff, SLTs, CAMHS workers or staff from local government/careers guidance initiatives. All avenues should be fully explored at a multi-agency review meeting.

Many parents talk of a particular individual or organization in the community that showed real understanding of SM and enabled their child to gradually participate and eventually shine in a particular area of interest or skill. As confidence and freedom of expression increased, there was a ripple effect into other social situations. We feel this is an area that has so far been relatively unexplored, with scope for investigating local opportunities such as charities, youth groups, clubs and volunteer agencies, with the aim of developing a local network of informed individuals and organizations who are willing and able to provide support to young people in the community.

Progress determined by improved social functioning

International consensus recommendations (Keen *et al.* 2008):

> The key criterion for considering that the child with SM is making progress is improved social function. This is demonstrated by an observable increase in non-verbal and verbal communication within a widening range of people and locations, accompanied by decreased social anxiety (as expressed by the child or evident through their demeanour).

The simple act of speaking is not an adequate measure of the child's progress towards being a spontaneous communicator who initiates interaction with others. There is a danger that 'she's talking now' can be reported and seen as progress away from the child's mutism, only to find that in fact the child is speaking under sufferance and quietly answering questions with a single word. This is not an indication that the child is any less anxious about the act of speaking or has become a more confident communicator.

In short, a talking child is not necessarily one that is communicating happily, freely and effectively. An ability to meet a widening range of communicative demands through non-verbal and verbal means is, however, a measure of success.

In keeping with the consensus recommendations, we note that checklists are being used to record not only who a child talks to, but whether the child can, for instance, gain a teacher's attention, express their need for the toilet, contribute to discussions, ask for help, report their experiences (such as unfavourable comments from others), or make choices at school lunch time. Does the child participate in group activities at school and in the community as a valued team member? Such information reveals as much about the knowledge and attitude of others as about the ability of the child to communicate, and provides a focus for education and intervention as well as a means of assessing and monitoring progress. Much of this is captured in the Selective Mutism Questionnaire (SMQ) (Bergman *et al.* 2008), which provides a measure of verbal communication and comfort in school, family and community settings.

The discharge criteria that accompany each care pathway are a clear indication that support services are using measures of social functioning to determine progress, as illustrated in Figures 11.3 and 11.4. It is a valuable exercise for services to identify discharge criteria in this way, recognizing that older children (late referrals) are likely to complete their recovery after discharge. Nonetheless, personal targets around participation and independence will be of greatest value to teenagers and give them a taste of what they can achieve with a fresh start in a new setting.

Access to a dedicated support group or organization

International consensus recommendations (Keen *et al.* 2008):

Educational and nursery (pre-school) professionals and parents should have access to the resources available from appropriate support groups (e.g. in the UK, the Selective Mutism Information & Research Association, SMIRA) as soon as SM is identified.

Given the relatively recent rise in interest and understanding about SM amongst professionals in health and education, parents are often left to their own devices when it comes to investigating and managing their children's mutism. Dedicated websites such as SMIRA are often their first 'port of call' and provide not only the vital information they need but also the peer support they were unable to find from friends and family. Even when parents are lucky enough to find local services with the time and expertise to support their child, many comment that it is the day-to-day access to internet chat-rooms hosted and moderated by organizations such as SMIRA that become their 'lifeline'.

We have found that services working with SM typically refer parents and other professionals to SMIRA via their training packages and advice leaflets. Group training sessions for parents have also provided a valuable forum for parents to share their experiences.

In conclusion

The SM care pathways in use and under development in the UK demonstrate a high level of consistency with the internationally agreed principles set out in 2008 by Keen, Fonseca and Wintgens. We recognize that each locality will vary in terms of which professionals are best placed to support children with SM, and recommend a flexible approach in applying the key principles as set out in Figure 11.5. Ultimately, we would like to see multi-agency care pathways in place so that every child with SM is steered without delay towards appropriate support, regardless of where the child lives and whom the family first approaches for advice. We hope this chapter will encourage readers to consider how they can become more involved in service provision for these children, regardless of their professional background and place of work, leading to collaboration between local services and organizations to agree a unified approach for recognition and management of SM.

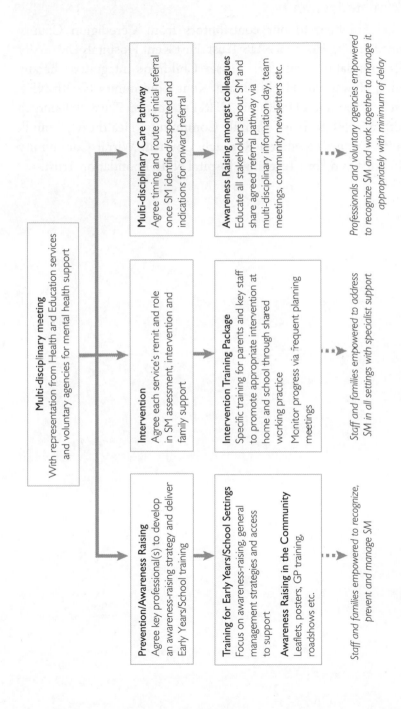

Multi-disciplinary meeting
With representation from Health and Education services and voluntary agencies for mental health support

Prevention/Awareness Raising
Agree key professional(s) to develop an awareness-raising strategy and deliver Early Years/School training

Training for Early Years/School Settings
Focus on awareness-raising, general management strategies and access to support

Awareness Raising in the Community
Leaflets, posters, GP training, roadshows etc.

Staff and families empowered to recognize, prevent and manage SM

Intervention
Agree each service's remit and role in SM assessment, intervention and family support

Intervention Training Package
Specific training for parents and key staff to promote appropriate intervention at home and school through shared working practice
Monitor progress via frequent planning meetings

Staff and families empowered to address SM in all settings with specialist support

Multi-disciplinary Care Pathway
Agree timing and route of initial referral once SM identified/suspected and indications for onward referral

Awareness Raising amongst colleagues
Educate all stakeholders about SM and share agreed referral pathway via multi-disciplinary information day, team meetings, community newsletters etc.

Professionals and voluntary agencies empowered to recognize SM and work together to manage it appropriately with minimum of delay

Figure 11.5 Multi-agency application of international consensus recommendations

Acknowledgements

We are indebted to our contributors from Ceredigion County Council, Ealing Hospital NHS Trust, East Kent Hospitals University NHS Foundation Trust, East Sussex Children's Integrated Therapy Service, Hywel Dda Health Board, Kent Community Health NHS Trust, Northumbria Healthcare NHS Foundation Trust, St George's Healthcare NHS Trust, Suffolk Community Healthcare, Suffolk County Council, Swindon Borough Council, Wirral Community NHS Trust and York Teaching Hospital NHS Foundation Trust.

CHAPTER 12

Approaches to Treatment of Selective Mutism in Other Languages

Alice Sluckin, Rae Smith, Nitza Katz-Bernstein and Keiko Kakuta

A case from Belgium

The following anonymized example shows how a child was helped within a very large Belgian school, without her parents having to exert pressure, because school staff were already familiar with the characteristics and needs of Selectively Mute (SM) children. Also, it appears to have been taken for granted that health and education staff would work together and include the family in any plans and that support would continue for as long as proved necessary.

A five-year-old trilingual, but SM, girl attended a Belgian school which has a proactive health policy. This meant that it has its own infirmary, approved health care workers including a contracted doctor, its own educational psychologist on the staff and, of course, Special Educational Needs Co-ordinators (SENCOs).

The school has 3000 pupils and uses 23 European languages, with many children becoming polyglot by the age of ten. However, it is accepted that children from minority language backgrounds, even in this unusually accepting environment, may be at risk for some delay in early language and that SM may increase that risk to some extent (Carmody 2000).

Several members of the girl's family had spoken freely at home but not at school – indeed, the family had their own nickname for such children – but they had not previously heard anything about SM, and found the diagnosis immensely helpful. They had observed their child's closed expression and protruding lower lip, but found the psychologist's comparison – 'a pressure cooker with the lid on' – 'a revelation'.

A letter about her diagnosis went to the school as well as to the family and the parents were advised to purchase Johnson and Wintgens (2001), which was described as 'a manual for teachers' and was in use as such with other children in the school.

After twice reading this book, the father constructed a detailed action plan with the school. This plan was granted 'approved' status, which meant that it was fully funded and was supported indefinitely by SENCOs, teachers and the school Director. Five years later, it is still in use to prepare for this child's transition to senior school.

Some treatment approaches in Germany

The treatment of SM children in Germany is mainly the responsibility of speech and language therapists and psychotherapists. In order to qualify for free services under the parents' insurance schemes, children have to be diagnosed by a medical doctor, who also has to recommend and oversee the treatment. This is usually of long duration, one to two years. Schools are involved in some regions, though not in all.

Mutism Self-help Germany

An organization founded, with Michael Lange, by specialist Speech Therapist Dr Boris Hartman is 'Mutismus Selbsthilfe Deutschland e.v.' ('Mutism Self-help Germany e.v.') www.mutismus.de, which both parents of SM children and SM adults can join (m.lange@mutismus. de) who organize meetings in different parts of Germany and sell very useful publications on the subject of SM (Hartman 1997, 2006;

Hartman and Lange 2005). They also publish a journal *Mutismus.de* and maintain close contact with British and American groups.

See also Mutismus Selbsthilfe Schweiz www.mutismus.ch in Switzerland.

Selective Mutism in children: an integrative approach

Here follows an account of the treatment method used by Nitza Katz-Bernstein, a highly qualified SLT/Psychotherapist based at that time in Dortmund, Germany.

INTRODUCTION: WHY AN INTEGRATIVE APPROACH?

Selective Mutism is a complex disorder and has an interdisciplinary character. In Germany and Switzerland there are some therapy approaches that are more behavioural, more systemic or psychodynamic (Hartmann 2006; Kramer 2006). At our Clinical Centre for Speech Disorders at the University of Dortmund, we developed and established the 'DortMut Approach' that presents an integration of all three approaches.[1] Our long-term experience showed that these children need specific approaches. The following factors indicate this:

- the complexity and interdisciplinary nature of the disorder between psychiatry, psychotherapy, speech therapy and special and/or integrative pedagogy

- the necessity of specific therapeutic media

- working with the (changing) resistance which is almost always present

- need for special handling of childish fears and ambivalence

- special concentration on speech therapy and language acquisition

---

1   Based on Katz-Bernstein (2013), www.fk-reha.tu-dortmund.de.

- necessity to combine interactive and psychodynamic oriented approaches

- defining the work with parents and co-ordinating the work with other professionals.

The therapy approach that I present here has a targeted integration of methods. Neither a non-directive play-therapy which pays little attention to the symptom, nor a strict behavioural programme can claim better efficiency if used as the sole approach (Dow *et al.* 1999). The various approaches and methods will be explained here in an overview.

THERAPEUTIC INTERVENTION: SOME PRINCIPLES WHICH MAKE THE DIFFERENCE

The quality of a therapy does not rely only on techniques, but also on the quality of the professional relationship (Miller *et al.* 2008). I can summarize the qualities as creating a 'holding professional frame' within the therapy:

1. Promoting self-reliance
2. Responsiveness to intentions:

    - assumption of a positive development

    - proximal approach (always requiring something 'in the zone of the next level of development' (Vygotsky 1978)

    - expanding tolerance of frustration

    - humour, playing with paradoxes, playfulness provocation

    - arousing motivation and curiosity

    - consistent adherence to common, declared limits

    - rituals, structure and demarcation of transitions

    - negotiating decisions about progress together

    - comfort and perseverance in the face of resignation, failure and errors, for example, 'Was it too soon? Maybe it was the wrong boy to be the first to speak to? Ah, we weren't paying attention. We must be more careful today!'

WITHIN THE THERAPY ROOM, MODULES OF INTERVENTION

How to build up basic communication?
Non-verbal steps

The 'safe place' is a therapy technique we use as a first step to build with the children, or, if not yet possible, to build for them a hiding corner, hut or tent, a so-called safe place within the therapy room while involving them in decisions about form, materials, size and so on, using the smallest bodily gestures or facial expressions to interpret their decisions. Usually they use the corner at the end of the first hour to hide, or hide the bear or the car they brought with them (Katz-Bernstein 2003, 2013), thus getting them to become involved and participate in a common interaction.

The strengthening of the 'alter ego'

Encouragement is a main part of therapeutic work. It includes the acceptance of the silence as a coping skill that also has a positive aspect and, as such, is not going to be 'taken away' by the therapy. The declared goal is to widen the possibilities for the child to decide freely whether to talk or not and ask if he/she wants to give it a chance. Usually it evokes an acceptance toward the next steps suggested.

The construction of a communicative
behavioural ability

This is a directive, at first non-verbal type of therapy (see Katz-Bernstein 2003). It initially includes building up pragmatic skills such as eye contact and exchange of facial expressions as well as using gestures to point, describe and illustrate objects, positions and feelings. All of these are implanted in a playful interaction, such as making a 'stop' gesture within a game.

WORKING WITH PUPPETS AND TRANSITIONAL OBJECTS

This usually works with smaller children. At first the child is only asked to be an observer. The therapist is speaking to the shy tortoise or to the snail, both very shy toward the new child entering the room. The therapist gently introduces the child to the tortoise, encourages it not to hide. Usually such a puppet becomes the best therapy assistant, beloved as a social model in how to co-operate, talk, become cheeky, etc.

BUILDING LANGUAGE WITHOUT SPEAKING

These activities are mainly for speech clinicians, based on some principles of the symbolic play of Pellegrini (2009). An interactive view allows the development of an interaction with a narrative. The therapist suggests a play context to the silent child, such as a bus ride with a driver and a passenger, or a take-away restaurant. This way the child can be involved in the events and gently enter into an interaction, first as a silent role-taker, later in dialogue and further interactions.

SYMBOLIZATION AND NARRATIVE PROCESSING: NARRATION WITHOUT LANGUAGE

Being trained as a psychotherapist allows a widening of the narrative possibilities for an intervention. In the sand-box, or by taking roles, the child will often tell us some of his narratives, usually being pursued by his (own) demands for perfection, fears of failure or even by real events of being abused. A psychotherapist who knows how to work with 'aggressive eruptions' will thus be able to socialize and 'tame' the aggressions in a symbolic-narrative way.

THE FAIRYTALE BOOK WITH SPEECH BUBBLES: 'HOWL, BOOM, SIGH…'

With school children, one child can play a wizard who can turn people into animals and then is asked to draw a picture of them interacting. Perhaps let them cut objects out of an old magazine – two that they like a lot and two which they find disgusting – while the therapist does the same; then they make a collage together. Once all objects are stuck down, the therapist suggests making some speech bubbles so these charcters can talk to each other, like comics. It seems to work as a transitional step to spoken words.

MODULES OF INTERVENTION: HOW TO BUILD UP SPEECH?

PRODUCING SOUNDS

As a first step with SM children, again, we are not talking yet but instead 'investigating the sounds in the room'. Usually silent children avoid producing any sounds at all. I offer an exercise where the child follows me, walking and knocking on different objects. After a while we change roles and I follow him, discovering new sounds in the room. This way eye contact, turn-taking and being involved in a structured way of interaction is established (Katz-Bernstein 2003, 2013).

FIRST WORDS

The first words I invent are a natural and obvious necessity within an actual interaction. For example, playing 'UNO': 'I think you can try and say UNO today! It makes it easier and is much more fun! I think it is going to work today.' If it didn't work, say: 'Don't let's give up. We cannot expect it to work immediately; we will try it again next time!' It is important for the therapist to stay supportive and encouraging. If it doesn't work, give the child a break: 'OK, today was the first try, often it takes time to get used to the idea / I am going to nag you next time / I hope that I don't annoy you by being like that.'

WORKING WITH A RECORDING DEVICE

To speak required items on a recording device (voices of animals, music played by the child, a role-playing game in a Mickey-Mouse language, even reading or telling stories with bigger children) is one of the well-known, successful ways of starting to talk. To let the child record noises – strange imaginative language sometimes, while I am outside of the room – is a very helpful strategy for bringing speech into the therapy room.

SHADOW SPEAKING AND FORCED MOVES

Some of the children seem to be able to talk when there is a 'shadow of noise' around them: playing rhythm with loud drums, playing certain music, saying things in a chorus of voices, shifting in a role-play, imitating noises of animals, machines, traffic, and talking some words.

HOMEWORK AND TRANSFER: HIERARCHY OF PLACE, PEOPLE AND WAY OF SPEAKING

As a next step I refer to the decision to increase freedom of speech as a contract, which I promise to fulfil. I say: 'Maybe it will be very easy for you and you will be astonished how it happens all by itself, or maybe it will not be so easy at the beginning, but we will just carry on.' As a first step, I let the child do some 'homework': 'You go to school and make a note of two teachers (children) you would like to speak to first and two of them you would like to be the last ones to talk with.' I regard this step as seriously as speaking the first word, but it is still easy, so I encourage the child: 'You see, you are doing well, the first step is done!' As a next step the child should say the answer to one question at school silently to himself, imagining he is doing so aloud, practising the real step within the therapy room. Later on we are going to invite his best friend to practise further. Step by step, we will later be inviting the favourite teacher to visit and discuss next steps and arrangements. We are going forward, never giving up!

THE END OF THE THERAPY

Evaluation will be made by the child, parents and teacher as to whether they all think the child doesn't need my support any more. A list of 'What I have learned', 'What I still want to learn', 'Some wishes for the future' and a celebration will signal the end of the therapy.

COOPERATION WITH FAMILY MEMBERS AND PROFESSIONALS

Working with parents of children, as well as the possibilities of working with teachers and social workers, medical and official professionals, is essential. This method, though, is child-centred, while the main goal is declared to be the widening of the communication skills of the child. The parents are usually not present in the room; they will be invited to attend special events – if the child so decides. That is the principle of the 'safe place'.

We will help parents, though, around the actual problem and questions arising, to strengthen their parental presence: to be supportive towards the child as 'the competent adult'. They learn to support their children to take some new steps and have some new experiences, in spite of their anxiety. Fear and anxiety are regarded as the old strategy that should be overcome (Lebowitz and Omer 2013) and the parents can learn to lose their own fear of the non-speaking behaviour of the child.

CONCLUSIONS

All these facets, techniques and suggestions are not meant to be seen here as additive and should not lead to a fragmented approach. The careful inclusion of both cognitive and emotional processes by the therapist ensures that the behavioural approach is founded on a psychodynamic, interactional and proximal approach. This is intended to help the individual components of the therapy to find a unifying and binding framework.

To summarize the approach above I will present four different approaches included in that concept for children with SM:

- sensitivity, empathy (psychodynamic approach)
- built-up co-operative actions (communicative approach)
- systematic training of communication and speech, transfer (behavioural approach)
- network (systemic approach).

All actions and approaches are based on resources and empowerment.

Current situation in Japan

We are grateful to Keiko Kakuta, representative of the Japanese Selective Mutism support group 'Knet' (abbreviation of 'Kanmoku network' – Selective Mutism Network with around 700 members) for producing this valuable account and to Kumi Andoh for translation.

Awareness of the needs of SM children seems to be at a fairly early stage in Japan. There is, as yet, little advice available for families, while school staff are not universally able to identify or respond sympathetically to children who fail to speak in class.

It was only around 2007 that the concepts of Special Needs Education and Individual Educational Needs started to be introduced into the Japanese educational system, so this should be taken into account, as well as other factors such as the school system and cultural background.

As teachers frequently deal with classes of 40 without assistance, it is difficult for them to do a great deal to help these most silent and least troublesome class members. In a normal class of a mainstream school, all are expected to perform in the same way, including pupils who may have some additional needs. Even though 6.5 per cent of children with a normal IQ showed noticeable academic and behavioural difficulties of various kinds in a government survey in 2012 (conducted by the Ministry of Education), 40 per cent of these children had never received any special educational support. This seems to indicate that services are in need of further development.

There are no official assessment systems for SM in Japan. Often, parents are informed by teachers or nursery nurses that the children are not talking. In many cases, they are just informed of their child's silence in school, not the fact that they are suffering from SM. Even if they use the term 'Selective Mutism', parents are often given misleading information such as, 'The child will grow out of it.'

By Japanese law, only doctors can perform a formal diagnosis. However, parents tend to seek advice from local organizations such as Child Consultation Centres and Child Development Support Centres, as well as having consultations with a school counsellor for school-age children. These centres give guidance and support for children's development under the state system. Assessments are mainly performed by psychologists or speech and language therapists who belong to the organizations, and these professionals may not have enough knowledge of SM. They mainly assess children's development by using IQ tests. Limitations are imposed by the practice of assessing only in the professionals' own places of work and by the difficulty of conducting formal assessments with a child who is not comfortable talking.

Since these organizations are independent of the school system, it is difficult for parents to organize a support team co-ordinating teachers and other professionals. In Japan it would be difficult for a parent to become a key-worker in school, since it isn't customary to have volunteers except for special activities. Although many schools provide a school counsellor or consulting services, the frequency and duration for each child doesn't seem to be sufficient.

Problems are apt to arise at school from time to time, as there is an expectation that all children will actively contribute in front of their class to formal speaking events and ceremonies. This type of activity presents SM children with a frightening challenge and one which their teachers' training does not equip them to recognize or ameliorate. Rather than teachers who express frustration and annoyance, SM children need teachers who will understand how to modify the demands of situations such as these.

Provision has been made in Japanese schools for intellectual impairment for a long time. Currently, there is provision for nine types of childhood special needs, including visual and hearing impairment, speech impairment, autism, emotional disorders and learning difficulties. Of these, SM is included in the category of emotional disorder. An SM child who has difficulties learning in a mainstream class might be enrolled in an SEN class or a short-term therapeutic institution for emotionally disturbed children.

For the last few years, some SM children have been able to attend special nurture groups known as 'Tsukyu' – held once or twice a week – with the aim of helping children to improve their social and academic performance. However, the provision of this service appears to be geographically uneven. School counsellors sometimes provide useful advice about not attempting to force SM children to speak, but there is little or no systematic behavioural treatment as there are currently very few professionals who practice Cognitive Behaviour Therapy (CBT) in Japan.

For the teachers themselves, there is no specific instruction or support around the topic of SM other than that provided by voluntary help groups or individuals, including Knet. Knet was formed by Keiko Kakuta, a specialist clinical psychologist, in 2007 – together with three parents of SM children. Through contact with Kumi Andoh, a well-informed learning support assistant, who undertook a good deal of translation, they made contact with SMIRA, whose handouts for professionals and for parents proved helpful. This network now has around 700 members and aims to tackle nationwide problems such as the shame and stigma surrounding SM, parental reluctance to ask for help, widespread misconceptions about the condition and lack of available treatment and training.

There is no SM specialist in Japan, although some research has been conducted since the 1960s. Although SM is commonly described as a rare condition with an incidence of 0.15–0.38 per cent in Japan (Kawai and Kawai 1994), the current true figure is unknown since a large-scale investigation has not been conducted in recent years. On top of this there are some problems with defining SM as there are confusions regarding judgement and co-existing disorders. It is noted by Keiko that some parents seem to be unaware of their children's slight difficulties in speech, language and communication mainly because of certain aspects and characteristics of Japanese language and culture.

Recently a specialist paediatrician, Dr Kanehara, conducted a detailed investigation of aetiology (causes) and co-morbidity (associated problems) in 23 children with SM aged 3 to 14 years old who attended his clinic. He reported that the co-morbidity rate was very high – 60 per cent were reported to have developmental disorder, of which more than 50 per cent had an Autism Spectrum Disorder (Kanehara *et al.* 2009, pp.169–171). However, nearly 74 per cent of these SM children initially came for consultations on account of co-existing developmental problems rather than SM itself, which may possibly have had an influence on the findings. More research based on the general population of SM needs to be conducted.

Depending on the nature of co-existing problems, a combination of emotional support, psychological therapy and gradual, step-by-step behavioural guidance seems to produce good results. Research projects to examine treatment options are now needed.

In February 2013, a dramatized SM story based on Kirsty Heslewood (who later became Miss England) was broadcast on prime-time television. This was the first major feature on SM in Japan and it has created awareness amongst the general public. Also, there have been more mentions of SM in newspapers recently, as well as more talks and workshops in conferences on children's developmental issues. This is due to the efforts by individuals and organizations such as Knet. We are hoping that these exposures and this awareness will lead to some kind of scheme in schools to deal with SM children in the near future.

CHAPTER 13

Music Therapy and the Path into Speech

Kate Jones

The case study in this chapter first appeared in the *British Journal of Music Therapy* (Jones 2012) and is reprinted here with permission.

Introduction

In this chapter I describe my experience of being a music therapist and researcher working in nursery and primary schools with children with Selective Mutism (SM). I then describe a case study of how music therapy helped a boy with SM. A theoretical framework describing how music therapy could help children with SM is then presented, explaining key features such as musical conversation, physical freedom, emotional communication and the creation of a path into speech.

Beginnings of a research journey

When I was first referred a child with SM, I had no awareness of the condition. Music therapists often encourage referrals of children with low levels of communication and try to ensure that they do not get overlooked in an education system where the louder children tend to receive more attention. Being referred children who are silent in school fits within our clinical expertise and knowledge. We find that these children often respond extremely well to music therapy intervention, sometimes within just a few weeks. This experience has motivated me to start a research journey to explore how and why this is.

My initial searches for information on SM revealed a significant history of thought and development of interventions in this area. Two publications, *Selective Mutism in Children* (Cline and Baldwin 2004) and *The Selective Mutism Resource Manual* (Johnson and Wintgens 2001), are invaluable resources for developing strategies to support children with SM. They also made me consider my role as a music therapist within a context where so much had already been achieved. The internet has also provided a wealth of information, resources and support for parents of children with SM. However, my investigations of these online discussion and support groups revealed a level of dissatisfaction among parents and children with SM with the degree of awareness and the availability of interventions for SM. The use of anti-depressant medication now appears to be widespread in the United States for young children with SM, although this is not yet the case in the UK where a behavioural approach is more common. If alternative treatments such as music therapy are shown to be effective, could these be offered within a multi-modal team approach?

Two articles (Amir 2005; Mahns 2003) are useful in their description of music therapy for children with SM and complex emotional issues, but neither really reflects my experience and approach to what seems to me to be such an obvious and pragmatic intervention for these children. Roe (1993) describes an interactive therapy group 'where all means of communicating – verbal and non-verbal – were accepted and encouraged' (p.134), which resonates more closely with my perspective. Providing an opportunity for being heard through free musical self-expression without the pressure of speech surely offers all the right tools to move into confident speech. Paths into SM have been described, but music therapy can perhaps provide a path out. In this chapter I set out to explore and identify a place for music therapy on the pathway into speech.

What is music therapy?

Music therapy is the use of music as a medium for self-expression, understanding and change within a supportive therapeutic relationship. Music therapists aim to create a space in which children can express themselves freely and feel that they are being listened to, heard and understood. Music therapy has very different aims from music lessons. The aim of a lesson is to teach, whereas the aim of therapy is therapeutic change – for example, self-expression, greater happiness, self-confidence, speech (Darnley-Smith and Patey 2003).

Music therapy sessions are often non-directive and so as music therapists we usually take the lead from how the child presents in the room and as far as possible allow them to direct the sessions. Children sometimes request specific songs or styles of music but mostly we use free improvization to develop musical conversations and musical 'play'. We often use a 'Hello' and 'Goodbye' song to help orientate children within the sessions. To help create a feeling of safety and 'containment', sessions should take place in the same space and at the same time each week.

I now briefly describe a case study of how music therapy intervention helped a child with SM.

Luis

Luis (not his real name) was a four-year-old boy with SM who was also learning English as an additional language by immersion only. He spoke another European language fluently at home and was referred to music therapy by his nursery school teacher who was concerned that he wasn't speaking at nursery after 10 months. It is usually thought that a 'silent period' of up to six months should be allowed for a child learning English as an additional language before speaking in school (Toppelberg et al. 2005).

Luis received 11 weekly sessions of music therapy of 30 minutes duration, provided by a not-for-profit music therapy service funded by the school and a local charity. The sessions took place in the music room that was situated close to his nursery classroom. Over the course of the therapy Luis moved from his nursery class into his reception class. This case study used 'meaningful moments' to tell the story of the therapy process. 'Meaningful moments' are those key events in the therapy sessions where something important seems to be happening or changing for the child (Figure 13.1).

1ST MEANINGFUL MOMENT – SESSION 4 – 00.00–07.00 MINUTES

This moment highlighted the first dramatic change in Luis. After three sessions of appearing to feel very anxious about therapy, there was a rapid development of musical engagement in the sessions. Here Luis played the xylophone with expressive, playful sweeping motions, arcing his arms in the air in dance-like movements. After playing music that aimed to provide a feeling of safety in the previous sessions, I now felt that he was able to tolerate more direct responses to his music such as turn-taking and some tentative eye contact. Luis then used the recorder (an oral instrument) and was gradually able to take part in a confident musical conversation that ended with the recorder being played pointing up in the air.

Luis then started rearranging the instruments in the room. This became a feature of subsequent sessions but began in this moment, with him creating a circle of instruments around him. He played them at first in rapid succession but then became more free, expressive and loud, using two hands. These were quite large, loud percussion instruments. It also felt significant that he was engaging with making a lot of sound after many months of silence within school.

2ND MEANINGFUL MOMENT – SESSION 4 – 29.00–32.00 MINUTES

This moment was chosen because it was the first time that Luis made use of a lot of language in the sessions. In session 3 he had said the single word 'toilet', but in this moment he pointed and spoke in a way that suggested he wanted to engage in verbal interaction. In this moment there was a lot of verbal turn-taking. Despite me not understanding some of his speech, it seemed important to engage in a turn-taking 'conversation', ignoring inaccuracies in order to allow speech to evolve naturally, without the speech feeling too pressured and too important.

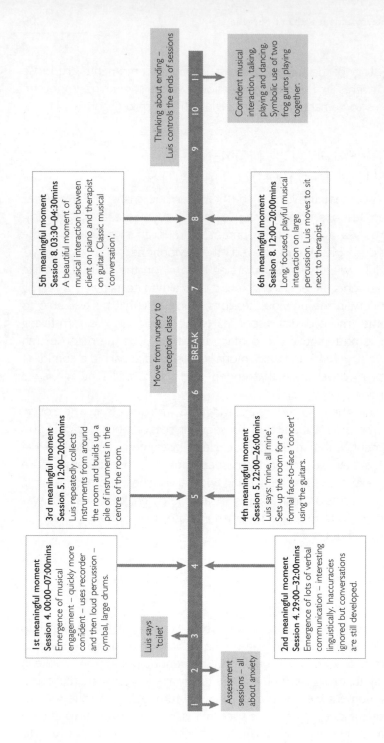

1st meaningful moment
Session 4. 00:00–07:00mins
Emergence of musical engagement – quickly more confident – uses recorder and then loud percussion – cymbal, large drums.

2nd meaningful moment
Session 4. 29:00–32:00mins
Emergence of lots of verbal communication – interesting linguistically. Inaccuracies ignored but conversations are still developed.

3rd meaningful moment
Session 5. 12:00–20:00mins
Luis repeatedly collects instruments from around the room and builds up a pile of instruments in the centre of the room.

4th meaningful moment
Session 5. 22:00–26:00mins
Luis says: 'mine, all mine'. Sets up the room for a formal face-to-face 'concert' using the guitars.

5th meaningful moment
Session 8. 03:30–04:30mins
A beautiful moment of musical interaction between client on piano and therapist on guitar. Classic musical 'conversation'.

6th meaningful moment
Session 8. 12:00–20:00mins
Long, focused, playful musical interaction on large percussion. Luis moves to sit next to therapist.

Assessment sessions – all about anxiety

Luis says 'tcilet'

Move from nursery to reception class

BREAK

Thinking about ending – Luis controls the ends of sessions

Confident musical interaction, talking, playing and dancing. Symbolic use of two frog guiros playing together.

1 2 3 4 5 6 7 8 9 10 11

Figure 13.1: Diagram of therapy

3RD MEANINGFUL MOMENT –
SESSION 5 – 12.00–20.00 MINUTES

This moment was chosen from the very next session and showed the quick succession of significant events in the therapy process. Before the session began, the nursery teacher had reported that Luis was 'coming out of himself' and that 'whatever you are doing, it is working'. Within the classroom he had produced some loud screams and used occasional single words.

In my session notes I reported that there seemed to be 'much less anxiety in the room'. The session began with some relaxed exploring of different instruments. The moment showed Luis repeatedly collecting instruments from around the room and building up a pile of them in the centre of the space. He gathered together keyboards, drums and boxes of small percussion instruments that he then tipped onto the instrument pile. He was happy and excited, and skipped and danced whilst collecting things. He vocalized 'ooh' excitedly and placed chairs in specific positions. Luis threw a cushion onto the pile, and then crashed some tambourines and cymbals on as well. This was all reflected by my sung commentary supported by a piano accompaniment that tried to match the happy but purposeful mood of the pile-building.

4TH MEANINGFUL MOMENT –
SESSION 5 – 22.00–26.00 MINUTES

This moment happened a few minutes after moment 3. I decided to move over to the drums and Luis responded to this change by going over to the guitars and beginning a conversation with me about them. It felt significant when he spoke the words, 'mine, all mine' in reference to another guitar that he was getting out. Luis' claim on the guitar and his sense of control and ownership of the therapy sessions seemed particularly important in this moment. The words 'mine, all mine' evolved into another quite extensive verbal conversation, again towards the end of a session. This time, however, it led into a formal 'face-to-face' guitar improvization, sitting on carefully arranged chairs. I commented in my notes that this felt like a concert.

5TH MEANINGFUL MOMENT – SESSION 8 – 03.30–04.30 MINUTES

This moment took place after the Christmas holidays when Luis moved from his nursery class into his reception class. Staff were concerned about how he would cope with this change and it felt important to show how the therapy developed after this transition. An initial conversation with his new teacher revealed her concern, when she described Luis as 'not talking generally at all, but he did ask to go out in the snow with his friend'. Given his low levels of speech in the nursery setting, this was actually a significant improvement for Luis. I communicated this to the teacher, but she felt that set against other children's normal speech Luis remained a concern for her.

This fifth moment was only a minute long and came near the beginning of session 8, the second session after the Christmas break. It was a moment of close musical interaction between Luis on piano and me on guitar. It can be described as a simple musical 'conversation', with intense, focused listening and clear musical reflection of his musical self-expression. The moment began with Luis playing a single note at the top of the piano and me responding with a high note on the guitar. He then developed a little melody on the piano that I again reflected on the guitar. Luis kept checking back and looking at me curiously to see how I would respond. There were more single-note interactions and then a longer descending melody initiated by Luis, closely followed by me reflecting the melody on the guitar. At the end of this intense interaction he moved to the window and pointed, saying 'outside'.

6TH MEANINGFUL MOMENT – SESSION 8 – 12.00–20.00 MINUTES

This moment occurred a little later in session 8 and was chosen because it was the longest moment of shared musical interaction in all the therapy sessions. I had set up the room with large drums and cymbals in the centre as this had seemed to fit Luis' musical preferences from previous sessions. Luis sat opposite me but was close enough to share some of the same instruments. The music and events were playful and free. He gave me some hand-bells that I then placed on the drum; eventually they fell off. He exclaimed in delight, accidentally hit the cymbal and then immediately afterwards he deliberately hit the cymbal. There was some 'same time' drumming (playing at the same time and stopping at the same time in a burst/pause sequence), which was directed by Luis.

Within these sessions I witnessed development in differing but connected aspects of the therapy. Parallel processes emerged that impacted upon each other and seemed to drive the therapy forward towards its positive outcome. These parallel aspects of the therapy process will now be discussed in the form of a theoretical framework.

Theoretical framework

The theoretical framework offers an explanation of the key elements of music therapy that are relevant in helping a child with SM (see Table 13.1 on following page).

TABLE 13.1 PROPOSED THEORETICAL FRAMEWORK FOR WORK WITH FOUNDATION-STAGE CHILDREN WITH SM

Therapeutic process	1. Offering a potential space	2. Manifesting anxiety – having it contained and processed	3. Gradual build-up of trust and contact through listening and accepting – 'no-pressure approach'	4. Gradual development of shared, meaningful communication and 'playing'	5. Need to end therapy – healthy, confident separation
Parallel layers of communication					
(a) Musical	Musical conversations – parallels spoken conversations – 'sliding-in'				
(b) Physical	Control and expression in the physical realm lead to control of the voice				
(c) Emotional/ social	Therapeutic relationship parallels mother/infant interaction = emotional/social communication				
TIME IN THERAPY →					

Parallel layers of communication

The parallel layers of communication – musical, physical and emotional – are the therapeutic tools of music therapy that are available in each session. These are illustrated below using the case study.

MUSICAL CONVERSATIONS: 'SHAPING' AND 'SLIDING-IN' TO SPEECH

A key therapeutic process was that of Luis developing musical 'conversations' just prior to using speech. This was seen in his clear turn-taking using an oral instrument (recorder) along with my vocal responses that made this closely resemble a verbal conversation at the start of session 4. A verbal conversation then happened at the end of session 4. That this conversation occurred at the end of the session is also pertinent, as this is often the time when people share the most important aspects in a therapy session. In this instance I felt the need to extend the session slightly, which gave Luis even more control over the therapy space. The use of his voice enabled him to gain more control over his environment and I felt that it was important for him to experience this sense of power and self-expression, which had been missing from his school life.

Behavioural techniques for children with SM often involve either the 'sliding-in' of speech from home into the school or 'shaping' – eliciting speech within school (Cline and Baldwin 2004; Johnson and Wintgens 2001). Music therapy provides a low-pressure intervention in the place that 'shaping' might be used. It creates a space for musical self-expression as well as a detailed understanding of the tools necessary to develop a clear path into speech. This music therapeutic path makes it possible for the child to 'slide in' from the medium of music and sounds into the medium of speech through the use of oral instruments, vocalizations and singing. The individually tailored music therapy approach allows each child to discover and create their own path to speech, at a speed that respects their accompanying emotional needs. That music therapy offers a space in which to make sounds and be heard is the first step down this path. The importance of being 'heard' and feeling 'listened to' in a previously threatening environment after an extended period of silence in that setting is intrinsic to the usefulness and efficacy of the musical therapeutic process.

The use of instruments in other ways is also noteworthy, as children with SM often head quickly towards the louder instruments (Roe 1993). The therapy path for some children can also be quite short and they may quickly move through from oral instruments to vocal sounds, or via non-verbal singing to words. That the path is often loud and short is perhaps a measure of the frustration and then relief felt by children with SM who 'can speak and want to speak, but don't' in the presence of certain people or situations (Johnson and Wintgens 2001, p.17).

Encouraging and supporting all vocal sounds enables the child to revisit the 'babbling' stage (Sylva and Lunt 1982) and, if necessary, to have the opportunity to develop confidence vocally before trying out actual words. Another child might 'slide in' by making very loud sounds with the instruments and make use of this volume of sound to disguise or cover initial trials at speaking. Other children will use different protective actions such as playing under a table or, like Luis, using words and instruments with their back turned to the therapist. In all these examples we can see how it is possible for a child to gradually move into speech whilst the therapist focuses on the musical communication, thus taking the pressure off the attempts at speech.

CONTROL AND EXPRESSION IN THE PHYSICAL REALM LEADS TO CONTROL OF THE VOICE

It is not uncommon for a child with SM to present as 'frozen' or physically restricted and therefore to have problems engaging with school activities such as physical education (Cline and Baldwin 2004). This idea was also understood and developed in the group work of Roe (1993), where children undertook physical activities in pairs in order to develop trust.

The importance of controlling the physical therapy space and of using dancing as another means of expression seemed significant for Luis. Being able to control instruments in a functional way, rearranging them and switching them on and off, seemed particularly important and symbolic, as SM can feel like a physical problem. Children with SM sometimes report later that they felt as if there was a physical constriction in their voice and throats.

The change in Luis' physical presentation appeared to signify and trigger a sense of liberation which began with his expressive xylophone playing (session 4) and then culminated in his dancing around the room collecting instruments (session 5). This sense of physical self-expression, control and ownership became core themes in the therapy as a whole. In session 5 this led to the emergence of verbal self-expression and the statement 'mine, all mine'.

THERAPEUTIC RELATIONSHIP PARALLELS MOTHER/INFANT INTERACTION: EMOTIONAL COMMUNICATION

Daniel Stern (2002) was interested in parent/infant interaction and described the function of early playful communication as primarily social and emotional using musical terminology. This provides a theoretical foundation for music therapy practice, where the development of a musical therapeutic relationship parallels this early parent/infant relationship. Within this therapeutic relationship it is possible to revisit and rework issues that arose at key developmental stages. For children with SM, music therapy offers them an opportunity to strengthen these communication skills through the use of musical self-expression within the setting that is causing them anxiety. With Luis, initially this was musical but it then moved into speech. As demonstrated in the case material, this focus on emotional communication is particularly relevant for SM where the therapeutic relationship can hold or contain some of the anxiety experienced by these children.

Therapeutic process

The therapeutic process is the emotional aspect of the music therapy that happens over the timespan of the intervention. The five stages in the process identified in the diagram are briefly discussed below in relation to the case study.

OFFERING A POTENTIAL SPACE

We know that children with SM can be extremely anxious and so finding the right space and developing rapport is crucial. The music room Luis and I used was very close to the nursery and so felt appropriate for a young child. Transitions were also important, and Luis and I spent a lot of time exploring frost, snow and puddles on our journeys to and from the music room.

CONTAINING AND PROCESSING ANXIETY

The role that anxiety plays for children with SM is crucial to acknowledge and think about in the therapy process. There are several issues that should be held in mind whilst developing an appropriate therapeutic approach:

1. Where has this anxiety come from?

2. Is it an extension of separation anxiety that has not been processed in the usual way through verbal self-expression and socialization in the nursery setting?

3. Is it social anxiety or simply anxiety about speech?

4. How can we reduce anxiety for this child?

Within the school environment the pressure of meeting educational targets creates anxiety for the teachers of a child with SM. This is then easily transferred back on to the child within the nursery. Luis' nursery teacher certainly wanted him to speak before he went up to his reception class and the pressure of the understandable expectation could well have affected Luis and unwittingly increased his anxiety further. This has also been my experience in other schools, where I have heard teachers saying to children, 'You have to speak before you go into reception.' It is important to acknowledge how genuine intentions to help a child with SM can be extremely detrimental.

Music therapists are trained to provide emotional and musical support for an anxious child. The therapeutic term for this is 'containment' or 'holding'. The role of containment is to acknowledge a child's anxiety whilst also creating a safe space for them to transform this anxiety through musical self-expression and play.

BUILDING TRUST AND CONTACT THROUGH LISTENING AND ACCEPTING: THE 'NO-PRESSURE' APPROACH

Carl Rogers' (1961) approach to psychotherapy refers to 'unconditional positive regard' or warmth in the therapeutic relationship, which seems completely in agreement with Johnson and Wintgens' (2001) 'no-pressure approach'.

In the first meaningful moment, Luis arranged the instruments in a circle around himself. This suggested a strong physical defence, and when Luis' improvization evolved it too became loud and strong. The anxiety he experienced in the first sessions resulted in a musical dialogue where we played with our backs turned to each other, which meant there was no possibility for direct eye contact. These all seemed to be examples of defence mechanisms against overwhelming communicative intrusions.

The role of defences was crucial to Luis' therapy process and can be viewed generally in SM work as an important protective strategy that needs to be treated respectfully in order to then build a trusting therapeutic relationship.

GRADUAL DEVELOPMENT OF SHARED, MEANINGFUL COMMUNICATION AND 'PLAYING'

Once the child has experienced this acceptance and trust, it becomes possible to move on and for the child to claim, own and then increase their participation in the therapeutic relationship. The therapy setting should then enable the child to express themselves in a variety of different ways. These can be musical, physical, emotional and verbal, as described in the first section of the framework.

Luis was able to extend his musical conversations in a more confident and deliberate way. The meaningful moments from session 8 exemplify this process, with the initial face-to-face, close interaction at the beginning of the session, followed later by an extended period of focused, shared music-making. As a result of this, Luis was then able to initiate and tolerate close musical connections, close physical proximity and face-to-face interaction. Humour also became an important feature of the sessions.

Significantly, after session 8 the class teacher said that she was 'really pleased as he is talking lots in class.'

NEED TO END THERAPY: HEALTHY, CONFIDENT SEPARATION

The process of separation and ending was important in that it reworked some of the difficult separation experienced when Luis first attended the nursery. However, this time there was a sense of a healthy child who confidently wanted to go back to class to generalize the verbal communication skills developed within music therapy.

The generalization of speech can be supported by chatting during the transition from the therapy room back into the classroom. The use of a friend in the therapy sessions can be another way of supporting a child who is finding it tricky to generalize their speech from the therapy room.

Discussion

The case study described above and the theoretical framework developed from that study have shown that music therapy has the potential to help a child with SM.

This was a single case study, and so multiple case study research would be needed to test how the ideas in this chapter can help other children with SM. If music therapy is accepted as a useful intervention, then where should it sit in the care pathway for children with SM? It is important to acknowledge that a multi-modal team approach is currently considered best practice and that any new interventions should be discussed as part of this team approach. Would music therapy also be useful for those children with a more complex presentation such as SM and Autistic Spectrum Disorder?

Music therapy seems to have the 'right tools in the toolkit' to help a child with SM and to create a bridge between home and the anxiety-provoking classroom environment. It offers a 'light touch' low-communication-load approach, with the focus on musical interaction rather than speech. The confidence that musical self-expression can bring leads to experimenting in ways that mirror and move down a path towards speech. Musical 'conversations', the use of oral instruments, the use of vocal sounds hidden beneath the sound of a cymbal, humming, singing and vocalizing are all examples of possible steps along this path at a pace chosen by the child. Most importantly, after a period of silence, it is a space to feel heard.

CHAPTER 14

Teaching Confidence to Teenagers

Rosemary Sage

Introduction

Can you think of times when you felt unsure of yourself? How did this affect behaviour? I remember crossing the road rather than having to talk to people I knew. My mum noticed this and signed me up for speech and drama classes. They were brilliant! The confidence gained has helped all aspects of life, underpinning my achievements.

Confidence is a powerful, elusive quality that creates success. Building this gives courage to try out different things. We normally approach new activities apprehensively, resulting in worry and confusion if problems occur. Persistence means we usually gain mastery, but if rescued by someone in the middle of an activity, we learn that they can do something that we cannot. In this chapter we consider what builds confidence, particularly for students in senior schools who experience communicative difficulties or consider themselves shy. First, consider the story of Ella.

Ella

Ella (not her real name) was a lively girl with three young brothers. However, when starting school she refused to talk. Her mum was beside herself and asked if she could join a Communication Opportunity Group (COG). This met weekly to have fun and encourage communication, based on narrative development (Sage 2000), assisting formal talk as in answering questions, giving instructions, re-telling experiences and making explanations. Children can chat well but have problems with formal classroom discourse. The first narrative level is generating ideas, so in a circle a box of objects is passed round and – when music stops – the one holding it selects something to talk about or demonstrate its use. Participants have an eight-hour programme, building narrative levels according to need. They then present five activities to help clarity, content, convention and conduct when communicating, for parents and friends, which are assessed for a certificate.

Although initially Ella responded non-verbally, when she felt confident she began to speak. She stuck with the group and now is a primary school teacher. She says: 'COGs coached me in things that were difficult. When I started school I was overwhelmed with talk and ducked out. I was shy, but now realize it was more than this. I couldn't make the move from home to class talk without help.'

What is confidence?

Put simply, it is the certainty that one is capable and can face life's challenges with awareness of self-worth. With confidence there is a realistic understanding of one's strengths and weaknesses, valuing the former and working on the latter. The socio-psychological concept of self-confidence is related to being assured of one's ability, judgement and power in any situation (Chandra 1999). It is having the attitude that – whatever the difficulty – one can handle it as well as possible. Also, one must appreciate that effort does not always bring immediate success. Do you know the story of the chap who developed Kentucky Fried Chicken (KFC) and knocked on a thousand doors before anyone would consider his product? Confidence in the future of this fast food was the driving-force that kept Mr KFC going. Being confident is infectious because it demonstrates power and control over people and events. If you come over well to others, they will want to copy your behaviour.

Arrogance, in contrast, is having unmerited confidence – believing something or someone is capable or correct when they are obviously

not. Overconfidence is excessive, unwarranted belief in something or
someone succeeding, without regard for possible failure. Confidence
can be a self-fulfilling prophecy. Those without it may fail, or not
try to achieve because they lack it; and those with it may succeed
because they have it, rather than superior, innate ability. Self-belief
is the driving force in behaving confidently and impressing others.

How confidence develops

Erikson (1963) describes the growth of confidence through
emotional development, in eight stages, influenced by the quality of
communicative relationships with other people:

1. Early infancy: trust versus mistrust

2. Late infancy: autonomy versus shame and doubt

3. Early childhood: initiative versus guilt

4. Middle childhood: competence versus inferiority

5. Adolescence: identity versus role confusion

6. Early adulthood: intimacy versus isolation

7. Middle adulthood: production versus stagnation

8. Late adulthood: self-acceptance versus despair.

The stages are based on a series of contrasts. As we go through life
we develop positive or negative concepts of ourselves in relation to
what happens and is communicated to us. So, if an infant has good
communicative relationships, she/he will learn trust, but if these are
bad, mistrust occurs (Sage 2000, 2007). Erikson proposes a growth
pattern of constructs which slot into learning. In school, when
children can compare performance against others, they grasp an idea
of their competence in relation to them. Seeing themselves doing
worse than peers means feelings of inferiority are experienced and
learned. Sage (2003) argues that these abstract concepts – based on
fundamental notions of good and bad feelings from events – are the
way children analyze the world. Early experiences – such as feeding

and care – generate positive or negative reactions from the child and are the measure for judging succeeding events.

Clearly, the concept of self that emerges includes children's overall view of their self (self-concept), body and abilities (self-image) and value (self-esteem). Self-confident people normally have high self-esteem. The earliest stage is the discovery that one is separate from others, constant and continuous. By age two, most children have learnt their name and, by three, achieved some autonomy because of physical, mental, social and emotional abilities. At four, a child shows possessiveness about space and things, and by five to six verbalizes thoughts and emotions and forms positive or negative judgements about theirself.

Much of self-image comes not only from what people perceive about themselves from daily experiences but from how they think others regard them. Therefore, they learn from others' reactions. Self-concept and values are affected by persons of significance in life – relatives, teachers, etc. So these adults must screen out those who pull down a child's character and encourage those that build it. A young person's self-concept comes from home and school nurturing, with peers being important as teenage years are reached. The deeper the roots of early self-confidence, the better equipped are children to interact with peers in a way that builds rather than destroys self-worth. They then know how to handle those who are amiable and others that are problematic. For healthy social development, children must first be comfortable with 'self' before they can be so with others. Being shy does not mean a poor self-image; it does suggest, however, that a child needs a boost to confidence, for adjusting to new situations and relationships and learning to be comfortable about interacting with others.

Baljit

Baljit (not his real name) was diagnosed with Elective Mutism and joined a communication group (COG) in school when aged seven years. The small group (eight students) and the interactive experiences (he particularly liked the mini-beast hunts!) helped him develop confidence and learn to communicate in a structured approach that gave him security, awareness and feelings of enjoyment and success.

Meadows (1993) reminds us, however, that children cannot be relied on to express feelings accurately, as it takes years to identify and communicate these explicitly. Also, many children have problems with communicating effectively in formal contexts such as school, because they lack the narrative thinking and language structures to understand and express ideas coherently with those that are unfamiliar. People with low esteem are anxious and struggle when coping with new situations. Others with high esteem have achievements valued and praised, experiencing a warm relationship with clear communication and limits set on behaviour (Merry 1998). Males are more confident in new tasks, but this may change as females take on more leading roles. It is important for youngsters to have opportunities to talk endlessly and observe and experiment constantly in a variety of situations so that they learn how to act and react. This happens in Japan, with schools the noisiest places imaginable, and students who are confident communicators can articulate their ideas, opinions and values.

Trying belatedly to impose values and ideas on a teenager – whose main developmental task at this stage is to identify their own beliefs – can be a difficult challenge. It is necessary, therefore, for parents and teachers to 'walk the talk' with a consistent model of behaviour to assist the social, emotional and mental development of those in their care. This is particularly difficult for shy parents, and those whose children have attended COGs have asked for help. This has been possible in several schools in Leicester, when teaching assistants have run COGs for students, their parents and in some cases grandparents, with great success.

Factors affecting self-confidence

Self-esteem has been directly connected to an individual's social network, the activities they take part in and what is communicated to them by others. Positive self-esteem has been linked to factors such as body image, physical and mental health, and mattering to those around them. In contrast, low self-esteem arises from a deprived background, poor relationships and communication, depression and antisocial behaviour such as bullying. Adolescents with poor health and wellbeing display low self-esteem.

If self-confidence is shaky, a youngster may view aggressiveness or bullying as normal, allowing themselves to be victimized or even making these behaviours part of their own. Children meet the challenge of new social groups with different behaviours. If they have a strong self-image, they are unlikely to be disturbed by them, but they might, however, become frustrated and experience stress which affects their emerging personalities.

Globally, self-confidence declines during adolescence. In contrast to males, it will not shoot up for females until early adulthood. The step from child to adult is a large one, with expectations of being independent both emotionally and economically. During adolescence, self-esteem is affected by body image, age, race, ethnicity, puberty, health, height, weight, physical prowess and attraction, gender presentation and identity as well as an awakening of sexuality. Adolescence, therefore, presents an opportunity for helpful intervention. Self-confidence, however, does vary according to personality and ability, and is observed in a variety of dimensions. For example, extrovert people come over as more confident than those who are introvert by nature. Components of social and academic life affect self-esteem. An individual's self-confidence can alter across contexts of both home and school, according to their feelings about these situations, and so contribute to a feeling of wellbeing or not (Myers, Wiliise and Villalba 2011).

The Wheel of Wellness was the first theoretical model of wellbeing, based in counselling theory, and has been used to support students in adolescence (Myers *et al.* 2011). It is based on Adler's individual psychology, together with cross-disciplinary research on characteristics of those living longer with a higher quality of life. Five life tasks are defined: spirituality, self-direction, work–leisure, friendship and love/regard. In the area of self-direction, further tasks are identified: sense of worth and control, realistic beliefs, emotional awareness and coping, creativity and problem solving, a sense of humour, suitable nutrition, exercise, self-care, stress management, gender and cultural identity. There are also five second-order factors: the coping, social, essential, creative and physical dimensions which allow exploration of the meaning of wellbeing within the total self. In order to achieve high self-esteem, it is important to identify strengths, positive assets and resources related to each component of the Wellness model, and use these to cope with life challenges. Factors in this model are reflected in the EU recommendations for key competencies necessary for the twenty-first-century citizen and researched by Sage (2011).

Implicit and explicit self-confidence

Implicit is defined as something implied or understood though not directly expressed. In contrast, explicit is something that is fully and clearly expressed with nothing implied. Implicitly versus explicitly measured self-esteem has been weakly correlated. Some experts, therefore, assume that explicit and implicit self-confidence are two different types of self-esteem. They conclude that one will either have a distinct, unconscious self-esteem or consciously misrepresent one's feelings. Studies have shown that implicit self-esteem does not specifically tap into the unconscious but that people over-report their levels of it. Another possibility is that implicit measurement may be assessing a different aspect of conscious self-esteem (Timko et al. 2010). Research also suggests that teachers have low expectations of some students, particularly for those with communication problems, with consequences for their self-value (Sage 2007).

Inaccurate self-evaluation is commonly observed even in healthy populations. Large differences between one's self-perception and actual behaviour indicate a number of disorders that have implications for teaching and the nature of interventions (Beer et al. 2010). Self-confidence does not necessarily imply a belief in being able to succeed in everything in life. For example, one may not be good at sport, music, drama or any other specific activity but still remain self-confident. This is the result of not placing too much emphasis on outcome, or being overcome by the negative consequences of something. It enables one to remain positive and self-confident by not worrying about failure or disapproval of others. One can then focus on the specific situation, so enjoyment and success is more likely. Belief in ability to perform successfully comes through positive experiences, adding to and consolidating self-confidence. This approach is the ethos of Japanese child-rearing and Sage (2012) shows how this leads to self-confident students who communicate well and are able to reach high levels of achievement.

Confidence in others

People can have confidence in other people or forces beyond immediate control. For example, one may have confidence in parents, teachers and police to protect and support. Sports fans have confidence that their team will win a game or top the league! Faith and trust are synonyms of confidence when used in this sense.

This is explained by conversion of objective evidence (observation) into subjective estimates (judgement). We mix true and false evidence during storage and retrieval of information to and from our memories (Hilbert 2012). Confidence biases results because we 'look inside our memories' (evaluate our confidence) and find evidence that is more extreme than when retrieved for making judgements (which are conservative due to mixing extreme values in the process). This explanation is sufficient to generate both overconfidence (in situations where judgement is sure) and under-confidence (in cases when it is judged that required knowledge is lacking).

How to build self-confidence at home and school

Confidence is built in oneself from positive support from others around. There are four major steps that can be identified in the process:

- Positive image results in self-confidence and depends on understanding one's own limits and trusting abilities. Those with a positive image can handle themselves in tough situations.

So, as teachers and parents, we must show confidence in young people and both verbal and non-verbal cues are important. I remember a teacher saying how lovely a student's picture was, but voice and facial grimaces showed otherwise! It is non-verbal cues that have most impact and being unconscious we need awareness of their negative impact on others.

- Acceptance results from complimenting what is done well. Try not to say 'You're good', but 'Luke, I liked the way you cleared up after work. You're good at organizing yourself.' Addressing by name – especially when accompanied by eye contact – conveys a 'you're special' message. Beginning interaction by using a name breaks barriers and softens corrective discipline. Also, being specific in what you say boosts confidence with useful feedback. If something is done inappropriately, comment calmly and quietly. It is important to say something like 'I appreciate that you've really tried.' Conveying the idea that without mistakes there is no learning or wisdom gained is vital! Suggest the 80/20 rule: no one is totally confident about everything. Be bold and confident about 80 per cent of the time.

- Encouraging initiative develops patience and confidence. In the UK we give students direct help in order to meet National Curriculum requirements. This encourages dependency and is in direct contrast to the Japanese approach when adults encourage trying rather than assisting students with tasks. It is important to be proud and positive of any response, so students will not fear new challenges and develop self-confidence to persist with tasks. Setting someone up to succeed avoids confidence being threatened. In our measuring and testing society, skills and their value are considered in relation to others. It is important to value the person for what they are rather than how they perform. Do this with plenty of eye-contact and focused attention. Reinforce that the one who achieves a skill first is often not the best in the long term. 'Probability goals', in a challenge, include an error margin:

'Let's see if you can get the ball into the net three out of ten throws.' This makes it less likely that someone will give up if they do not succeed first time. It is necessary to convey belief that the challenge can be met and that mistakes are the only way to improve.

- Act as a role model, as others learn most from your behaviour. Both parents and teachers are observed and imitated as significant people in youngsters' lives. Children copy adults to be like them. If they see you helping others, they will try to do so too. Requesting assistance from them when appropriate communicates regard for their capability and competence, and builds self-esteem. However, if they hear you talking negatively about people and things, they will do so too and believe the same might be said about them at some time.

Such steps depend on knowing and understanding students well, treating them always with respect, and giving unconditional, positive regard and support. This requires masses of positive reinforcement, providing boundaries and advice and instilling direction and realistic goals to be achieved in small steps. If you can help someone to think confident, they will be confident, with doubt eliminated and lifelong self-esteem promoted. Obviously, one cannot completely protect the young from the unpleasantness of the world, or shield them from unkind peers. However, they can be built up, strengthened and supported as they move towards complete independence.

Issues regarding specific communication difficulties

This book is about people who talk in some circumstances but not in others. According to your educational and training background and experiences, you will have a particular perspective on this situation. Typically, those who display this behaviour talk normally with familiar people, but clam up in less familiar circumstances such as school. Some experts consider this as extreme shyness and largely a mental heath issue. However, others suggest there is a problem moving from informal (chat) to formal (informative) styles of communicating. Informal talk does not have a planned outcome to the exchange and is highly interactive, with participants sharing responsibility for topics. The talk can progress in any direction but there is mutual understanding of what is expressed. This conversation is typically mundane about common routine experiences and events, requiring little analytic activity and opportunities to control the situation (Wood 1999).

In contrast, class talk is formal and directed to particular goals with emphasis on technical terms and word meanings, and less opportunity to control events. It is mentally complex, demanding the processing of large quantities of information, remote from individual concerns, frequently referring to a context not normally present. Also, most talk in schools is directed to groups rather than individuals. This requires assumptions to be made and a discourse level with many questions and commands that are unfamiliar to most children. Learners need to put together information and explain things, as in responding to 'How' and 'Why' requests. Research shows that many students leave school without formal communication competencies to cope with life and work (Sage 2012).

To succeed in the classroom, students must understand the specific ways to use language and communication in a relevant, appropriate manner. This requires them to judge what they do and modify this if indicated on another occasion. Many students do not develop this awareness of the different requirements of language until relatively late. Sage (2000) goes into this issue of home and class talk in some detail, with findings that provide evidence that this shift between discourse levels is not always understood by educationalists. Children can converse adequately informally but be completely flummoxed when faced with formal talk situations. This suggests how important it is for them to be given opportunities to practise formal communication activities, as this is the foundation for co-operating, collaborating and learning with others.

A Communication Opportunity Group Strategy (COGS) has been particularly successful in building formal language competencies and has worldwide endorsement in recent development studies undertaken by teachers studying with the College of Teachers (TCOT). Courses are now available for any interested person online at reasonable prices.[1] In this chapter it is not possible to expand on this approach but information is readily available from TCOT, which resides in the Institute of Education in London. To reflect on what has been discussed and to review your thoughts and opinions, have a look at the suggestions to generally help confidence and communication in the section below.

Here is a random collection of suggestions to boost confidence in others, which has been collected from friends and colleagues. Can you put them in rank order as to what you regard as most to least important?

- Encourage others to develop strategies for tasks, resisting providing solutions.
- Comment on achievements positively and reinforce appropriate behaviour.
- Encourage others to build a support network, identifying who can help them.
- Give tasks that can easily be done, giving value and importance to these.
- Show an interest in their lives and experiences, discussing problems together.
- Reinforce personal safety principles – it is OK to say 'no' for self-protection.
- Encourage others to trust feelings and share what is fearful or hurtful.
- Respect privacy and a need for personal space.
- Suggest that you are available when needed for anything.
- Give others responsibilities and reinforce their value.

---

1   See www.collegeofteachers.ac.uk/Learn

- Laugh *with* others not *at* them, showing regard and respect at all times.

- Say 'sorry' if you have made a mistake and encourage others to do so.

- Point out that mistakes are natural to growing and learning.

- Talk with, rather than at, others, smiling happily to be interacting with them.

- Be consistent always, and if others misbehave, they are OK, but not their behaviour.

- Consult over decisions to involve everyone in the process.

- Focus on a need to care for oneself, relax and enjoy experiences.

- Be calm and fair, refraining from imposing your thoughts or attitudes on others.

- Avoid nagging and bullying.

- Ensure that your verbal and non-verbal behaviour match in interactions.

Final thoughts

You cannot make others feel confident. Security and insecurity are functions of the self. However, it is perfectly possible to help them to find confidence, assuming they want to achieve it. Confident people dare to do things, take calculated risks, learn from experiences and are willing to take on new challenges and enjoy them. Confidence takes them through life successfully and allows failure to be coped with positively – it is the result of risk-taking. Reviewing times when students have achieved something well helps to build self-worth by acquiring self-awareness and self-respect.

Self-confidence is defined as having a realistic idea of one's own judgement, ability and power. It is a belief in an ability to succeed with an 'I can' rather than an 'I am' response. Teenagers who are confident grow up to have a positive sense of self and become balanced adults.

Parents and teachers can help them build confidence through adolescence, and this chapter gives some ideas for reflection.

Teenagers today consume vast quantities of junk food. They take many risks and do not really care about health and safety. It is the nature of this stage in life, but parents and teachers can encourage them to be healthier, more aware people who can withstand life's hard knocks. We can help others to develop self-confidence by encouraging them to:

- know the facts of a situation to make sensible judgements
- be ready, anticipating others' behaviour and preparing responses to this
- prepare well for situations, using open questions to assert and control
- practise for reactions with positive mantras, written to be often read (I will not be put down; I can do it; I will not let others upset me; etc.)
- have faith in abilities and personal style which will work if you let them
- feel sympathy/empathy for bullies – they need it!
- take note of things that inspire and reinforce proper values and attitudes
- be aware of your own strengths and weaknesses and plan for self-development
- relax and enjoy experiences to keep a perspective and balance to life
- never be afraid to take calculated risks as this is the key to progress.

Beliefs make the difference between confidence and a lack of it, understanding they are only opinions and not facts. Inaccurate or biased beliefs can be changed. We all hold particular views on why people can talk in some circumstances and not others. It is likely to be a blend of causes that are both communicative and psychological. Confidence is rooted in communicative ability and relationships that evolve from this. A lack of confidence alone is not a recognized mental heath issue but will impact on this. Holding negative beliefs about oneself lowers resilience and ability to cope with life stresses. This places people at a higher risk of developing problems such as social phobias or depression related to mood and self-belief. They then find that pressure of other symptoms such as a communication problem impacts on the way they view themselves.

The consequences of a lack of confidence, low self-esteem and communication difficulty are significant in all areas of life and can confirm a view of being of little value. They influence personal relationships with feelings of not deserving love and respect, so allowing others to take advantage and control situations. It can be difficult, therefore, to hear criticism and receive it constructively. This results in being oversensitive and easily upset, so situations and activities requiring judgement are avoided, leading to isolation and frustration. If lack of confidence and communication come from a belief of limited competence and intelligence, work will be a struggle and difficult tasks not attempted.

Teenagers need an extra boost to their self-confidence as they step up to adult responsibilities, and a COG came up with ten tips to help themselves which are well worth sharing and help summarize this discussion. These are:

- Never put yourself down.

- Make a habit of saying good things about yourself to yourself.

- Be helpful and considerate to other people.

- Become aware of things you are good at.

- Make friends with those who support you.

- Pursue work and interests that are interesting and enjoyable.

- Learn to be assertive and not allow others to put you down.

- Value your communication and aim to extend and improve it.

- Stop comparing yourself to other people – you are unique!

- Understand life has ups and downs and find ways to survive the latter.

CHAPTER 15

Legal Issues in Selective Mutism

What Support is a Child Entitled to?

Denise Lanes and Rae Smith

Parents or guardians who are seeking help for a child who is consistently silent in certain situations but not in others may find it helpful to remember that they and the child have certain rights under current UK law – for example, the Equality Act (2010) or the Children and Families Act (2014). This may mean, for instance, that if a 'Disability' or 'Special Educational Need' has been specified, there are certain absolute entitlements for which your child may qualify. It is worth keeping in mind that a House of Lords amendment to the bill ensures that, in the Children and Families Act itself, Speech and Language Therapy remains an educational need. In other words, SLT is not entirely dependent upon 'Health' funding, despite any misleading statements to the contrary.

For legal purposes, it is essential for Selectively Mute (SM) children to have a firm diagnosis. This is because it is easy for uninformed people to assume that they are simply being unco-operative. SM is now officially classified as a disabling anxiety disorder (APA 2013; WHO 1999, updated).

To be diagnosed as 'Selectively Mute', a child must be consistently silent in some situations, but speak freely in others, usually at home; have attended school or nursery for more than one term; and been immersed or instructed in the dominant language for more than six months. The fact that there may be co-existing conditions or a variety of causes should not rule out a diagnosis of SM.

Some families with SM children will be involved in a productive partnership with the child's school, working together to meet his or her needs. Some will receive support and intervention via the special educational needs (SEN) provision in their school or at home via Community Health. The school, or clinic, in partnership with the parents, understands the child's needs and provides appropriate support. Assessment by a speech and language therapist and an educational psychologist is arranged by the school or Child and Adolescent Mental Health team to inform this provision.

For other families, the situation is very different and this chapter has been written to inform those parents of their child's rights under current UK legislation.

The first recourse for parents is to try to negotiate support for their child via their GP (general practitioner) or the SEN process in school. There is now a revised Code of Practice recommending how children with SEND (Special Educational Needs and Disabilities) should be helped within the educational system. As the code has changed, it will be useful to understand its important features and to know where to seek help in navigating the new system.

The new Act comes into force in September 2014. However, its implementation will be subject to adjustments in practice. This will mean that parents are expected to put forward the case for individual children who do not have Education and Care Plans receiving any help they require.

The SEND Code of Practice provides statutory guidance on duties, policies and procedures relating to Part 3 of the Act and associated legislation and regulations (e.g. the Equality Act 2010).

A copy of these two important documents can be obtained from the following websites:

- Children and Families Act 2014: www.legislation.gov.uk/ukpga/2014/6/contents/enacted

- SEND Code of Practice 0–25: www.gov.uk/government/publications/send-code-of-practice-0-to-25.

In this new legislation, the definition of special educational needs has changed slightly. The new definition states:

> A child or young person has SEND if they have a learning difficulty or disability which calls for special educational provision to be made for him or her.
>
> A child of compulsory school age or a young person has a learning difficulty or disability if he or she:
>
> - has a significantly greater difficulty learning than the majority of others of the same age; or
>
> - has a disability which prevents or hinders him or her from making use of facilities of a kind generally provided for others of the same age in mainstream schools or mainstream post-16 institutions, including academies, special schools and free schools.

This second category may apply to children with SM if serious anxiety disorders prevent them from speaking at school.

To summarize, the major legislative and statutory changes include:

- Statements will be replaced by Education, Health and Care Plans (EHC). EHC plans will provide statutory protection comparable to statements. They will extend to age 19, whether or not the young person is at school.

- Consideration of Special Educational Needs will last until the age of 25.

- Health Services and the Local Authority will jointly commission and plan services as part of the EHC plan. Usefully, a 'designated medical officer' in the commissioning process can also be a 'designated clinical officer', for instance an SLT or psychologist.

- Parents and young people over the age of 16 may be given funding to purchase services identified on their EHC. However, it is expected that in reality the use of personal budgets will be limited.

- Local Authorities will publish a 'local offer', describing provision for pupils with SEN in their area.

- School action and school action plus will be replaced by a graduated approach.

- In due course, schools will also be required to publish their own SEN offers.

- Greater responsibility than before will be placed upon schools, therefore what they provide will inevitably vary.

- Quite complex arrangements for dealing with disagreements will be in place enabling both parents and older children to put forward their views and expectations.

For an analysis of the proposed changes, the following public service and voluntary organization websites are very useful:

- IPSEA (Independent Panel for Special Education Advice): www.ipsea.org.uk

- Public Service Info: www.publicserviceinfo.co.uk

- The Communication Trust: www.communicationtrust.org.uk.

It may not always be clear exactly who is responsible for funding these recommendations and ensuring that they are met. Families in some areas of the country may need to press quite hard for assessment and treatment, and for proper information to be made available to all the professionals involved with their SM child.

If an SM child is denied appropriate support via SEND pathways, there is powerful recourse for parents through an Act of Parliament described below. Parents will need to agree to their child being described as having a disability, which can be a difficult step to take. Also, the struggle to establish their child's right to appropriate intervention can be emotionally draining, but the rewards can be great. The child's school benefits too, with regard to better understanding of SM and wider disability issues. The definition of a disability in the Act is: a physical or mental impairment which has a substantial and long-term adverse effect on their ability to carry out normal day-to-day activities. This includes learning difficulties, mental health conditions, medical conditions and hidden impairments such as specific learning difficulties, autism and speech, language and communication impairments. Prevention of increasing disability is often the aim of treatment.

Since it is frequently assumed that SM children are voluntarily withholding speech, the supporters of selectively mute individuals may need to explain that many of them become physically unable to speak, or may feel so terrified of speaking that even trying to do so is impossible. That is the explanation for an apparent refusal to speak in some cases.

Young people of secondary age and above have a legal entitlement to complain themselves if they are discriminated against or are not provided with services that help them to overcome disabilities. Mina in Chapter 16 did exactly this by writing to the mentor at her school and obtaining the help she needed to overcome her SM as she wished to do. Had this failed, she could have taken matters further.

Below, we outline relevant aspects of the Equality Act that parents and children can use to obtain suitable provision for their SM child, together with contact details of useful organizations.

The Equality Act (2010)

In October 2010, this Act replaced all existing equality legislation, including the Disability Discrimination Act (2005). As SM is categorized as an emotional disorder related to severe anxiety, it falls within the categories covered by this law. The term 'protected characteristic' is used as a convenient way to refer to categories covered by the law.

The Equality Act Guidance of February 2013[1] has been compiled to help, for example, schools and parents to understand what is covered under this important law. Chapter 4 of the Guidance is particularly relevant as it outlines schools' responsibilities under the law, now incorporated in their SEND Code of Practice. These responsibilities are summarized here.

---

1 This can be found in full at www.gov.uk/equality-act-2010-guidance.

There are five kinds of unlawful behaviour that schools must avoid:

- *Direct discrimination.* This refers to the most obvious and clear-cut discriminatory behaviour. For example, an SM pupil fails to answer the register after repeated requests and is given a detention.

- *Indirect discrimination.* This occurs where a provision, criterion or practice is applied generally but has the effect of putting people with a particular characteristic at a disadvantage when compared to others without that particular characteristic. For example, a school uses oral group work to help pupils enhance their understanding of a topic by exploring meanings of key concepts, but the SM pupil is unable to participate without help that is not made available.

- *Discrimination arising from a disability.* A school must not discriminate against a disabled pupil because of something that is a consequence of their disability. For example, failing to assess and track an SM pupil's reading attainments, due to the method used in the school to assess reading (which involves reading aloud in class).

- *Harassment.* This is defined as unwanted conduct related to a relevant, protected characteristic. A school must not harass a pupil because of her/his disability. For example, a teacher shouting at a pupil because the disability means that s/he is constantly struggling with certain types of classwork.

- *Victimization.* This occurs when a person is treated less favourably than they otherwise would have been because of something they have done (a 'protected act') in connection with the Act. A 'protected act' may involve, for example, making an allegation of discrimination or bringing a case under the Act. Also, a child must not be victimized because of something done by, for example, their parents, in relation to the Act.

So what is expected of schools with respect to the law?

1. Schools must make reasonable adjustments:

    (i)   Where something a school does places a disabled pupil at a disadvantage compared to other pupils, then the school must take reasonable steps to try and avoid that disadvantage.

    (ii) From September 2012, schools are expected to provide auxiliary aids and services for a disabled pupil when it would be reasonable to do so and if such aids would alleviate any substantial disadvantage that the pupil faces.

    (iii) Failure to make reasonable adjustments can no longer be defended as justified.

The Equality and Human Rights Commission (EHRC) has published guidance on the auxiliary aids duty.[2]

2. Schools must implement accessibility plans which are aimed at:

    (i)   increasing the extent to which disabled pupils can participate in the curriculum

    (ii) improving the physical environment

    (iii) improving the availability of accessible information to disabled pupils.

3. Schools must meet the Public Sector Equality Duty (PSED). Schools must show that they have due regard for the need to:

    (i)   eliminate discrimination and other conduct as prohibited by the Act

    (ii) advance equality of opportunity between people who share a protected characteristic and people who do not share it

    (iii) foster good relations across all characteristics

---

2   It is available at: www.gov.uk/government/publications/equality-act-2010-advice-for-schools.

    (iv)   ensure that decision-makers in schools are aware of the duty to have due regard to the Act when making a decision or taking an action

    (v)   consider equality implications before and at the time that they develop policy and take decisions.

The PSED has to be integrated into the carrying out of the school's functions. It must not be a tick-box exercise.

4.   Schools must:

    (i)   publish information to demonstrate how they are complying with the PSED

    (ii)   prepare and publish equality objectives.

This information needs to be updated at least annually and objectives published at least every four years. The simplest way for schools to publish this information is to set up an equalities page on the school website. It must be accessible to the school community and to the general public.

Responsibility of Local Authorities

Local Authorities are under the same duty as schools:

- to have accessibility strategies
- to provide reasonable adjustments
- to provide auxiliary aids and services.

Discrimination claims

Specialist tribunals with experience and knowledge of disability issues hear cases of contravention of the educational provisions on the grounds of disability.

If a tribunal finds in a pupil's favour, the remedy will be with a view to removing or reducing the adverse effect on the pupil concerned. There is no financial compensation. However, schools may have to allocate funds to remediate the issue.

The 'questions procedure'

A pupil (or someone representing the pupil) can ask questions of the school before deciding whether to bring a case. There is information about this procedure on the website of the Equality and Human Rights Commission.[3]

If there is no response to these questions from the school after eight weeks, or the answers are vague or evasive, a subsequent tribunal can draw an adverse inference from this.

International conventions

The legal position is further strengthened by means of two international conventions, as described below.

The United Nations Convention on the Rights of Persons with Disabilities

On 23 December 2010, the European Union ratified the UN Convention on the Rights of Persons with Disabilities. Ratification means that EU is now bound to ensure that the rights of persons with disabilities are respected, protected and fulfilled. Furthermore, recent decisions of the European Court of Human Rights have broadened the scope of protection for people with disabilities.[4]

It will be useful for parents to remember that from 2007 educational establishments in the UK have a responsibility to consider the social and emotional development and wellbeing of pupils (i.e. their mental health), in addition to their inclusion, access to the curriculum and academic progress (DFES 2007).

Where SM is concerned, this involves ensuring that all staff become well informed about the condition, and in particular the adult attitudes and behaviours that are likely to make it worse. Staff should also be aware that treatment is possible and best put in place at an early age.

---

3   Available at www.equalityhumanrights.com/advice-and-guidance/education-providers-schools-guidance.

4   For further information, visit www.equalrightstrust.org.

The fact that neglecting an obvious communication difficulty can be damaging to a pupil's academic, social and emotional progress is becoming well understood. However, it can go unnoticed that mute youngsters, who seem to comply peacefully with the demands of school or college life, can be in serious danger of similar neglect.

The European Convention on the Rights of the Child

Certain rights apply to everyone under the age of 18. The Convention, adopted by the UK in 2008, specifies, among many other rights, those of children to:

- say what they think should happen, when adults are making decisions that affect them and to have their opinions taken into account (article 12)

- get and to share information, as long as that information is not damaging to them or to others (article 13)

- be protected from violence, abuse and neglect (article 19)

- receive special care and support if they have any type of disability, so that they can lead full and independent lives (article 23)

- receive legal help if they are accused of breaking the law (article 40).

Governments should make the Convention known to parents and children (article 42).

Duty of care

As shown in this volume, 'selective' or 'situational' mutism can happen for a number of reasons, few of them under a child's voluntary control. For this reason, a variety of professionals who may be in a position to provide assistance could be said to have a 'duty of care' toward children thought to suffer from the condition. In present circumstances, however, it is not clear whether sufficient scientifically validated information is available to all professionals who might be liable or whether the services in which they operate have the capacity to include these children in their remit.

What is clear is that:

- selectively mute behaviour can and should always be identified by teachers and nursery nurses

- speech and language therapists can and should fully assess all aspects of communication ability in children thus identified by visiting their homes or obtaining reports and recordings from parents or guardians

- a variety of treatment approaches appear to have potential and require further investigation by a number of different professional groups.

The criminal justice system

Children as witnesses

Children who are required to appear as witnesses in criminal proceedings seldom find this an easy task. Support is now always available for minors. In the case of children with any type of speech, language and communication needs, specialist support is available and families can insist that this is arranged. Court appearance would be highly likely to feature as one of the situations that a selectively mute child would find inhibiting. For this reason, such a child might need to give evidence in an unconventional way. A method would need to be devised imaginatively by a supporter who thoroughly understood the condition.

Children who may have committed a crime

A selectively mute child accused of a crime would be in an especially difficult position. It seems likely that his or her silence would be interpreted by most adults as voluntary and therefore an indication of guilt. In a situation like this, there would be an absolute necessity to involve a specialist practitioner who could devise methods of responding and explain that, although guilt could be a reality, the accused's silence is likely to be be attributable to an anxiety condition formally recognized by the Royal College of Speech and Language Therapists, *DSM-5* and *ICD 10*.

Voluntary organizations supporting families

- Independent Panel for Special Education Advice (IPSEA) www.ipsea.org.uk is a long-established organization with an excellent reputation. It has an advice line, advice on 'how to take action', and a tribunal helpline (Tel. 0845 602 9579).

- Advisory Centre for Educational Advice (ACE) Education www.ace-ed.org.uk is another long-established organization offering advice on special educational needs and disability discrimination (Advice line: Tel. 03000 115 142).

- Afasic www.afasic.org.uk (Advice line: Tel. 0845 355 5577 or 0207 7490 9420/9421).

- Parent Partnership is an organization in each Local Authority, funded by LAs but independent of them. All schools should be distributing Parent Partnership leaflets outlining the local service, which includes information about LA arrangements for SEN, and representation at school and LA meetings when required.

- Special Needs Jungle www.specialneedsjungle.com

See in addition:

- Government guidance *The Parents' Guide to the SEN and Disability Reforms*, which can be accessed on https://www.gov.uk/government/publications/send-guide-for-parents-and-carers or requested as a paper version.

- There is also a useful app produced by the Council for Disabled Children to enable families and young people to store, organize and share information about them and the support and services they receive, available at www.councilfordisabledchildren.org.uk/what-we-do/networks-campaigning/early-support/early-support-app.

PART IV

Conclusion

CHAPTER 16

Recovery from Selective Mutism

Testimonies from Families No Longer Affected by SM

*Alice Sluckin, Katie Herbert, Mina Clark
and a SMIRA Parent*

Katie's story

Katie (not her real name) and her mother tell the story of her troubles and eventual recovery in their own words.

My Mum recalls how I was always more reserved than other children – even as a baby I was less adventurous than others. When other parents were talking about how they were always running after their children who just wanted to explore, my Mum would always look down and see me by her feet, scared to leave her side.

I somehow had a fear of people outside the family; at home I was fine but as soon as other people were around things would be different. Obviously I had to go to school though. Some children would cry and try and resist being left but instead my whole body just became numb and my face blank. I didn't want to be there but just accepted I had no choice. I just went through the motions but it would be like I wasn't really there. My Mum noticed how I would be really chatty on the way to school and then at a certain point I would just automatically change.

To me, it was natural to be quiet and to retreat into my own little shell. I just remember being so overwhelmed by all these noisy children who wanted to be the centre of attention all the time when I just wanted to sit back and watch from the sidelines.

Mother speaks: Katie always seemed happy and relaxed at home or with people she was familiar with and felt comfortable with but was noticeably different in unfamiliar situations. She particularly seemed overwhelmed by playgroups or school. She didn't cry but seemed resigned and braced herself. I could tell how tense she was, almost robotic, paralyzed with fear. We hoped she was just shy and would adjust eventually. It wasn't until I talked to her Year 1 teacher about how unhappy she was at school that she informed me that actually in two terms she had never heard her talk!

Plans to help her integrate and speak in small groups never seemed to be put into action. I did think of asking for professional advice but wasn't sure who to ask and was concerned about making Katie feel more anxious by being singled out. I was also very aware of the potential for her not talking at school being misunderstood. It broke my heart to see her so isolated and occasionally I would see the same frightened rabbit look and inability to speak in other situations. By the time Katie was five she had three younger siblings and her mutism at school began to become entrenched.

With hindsight I wonder if my inability to help or understand left her feeling abandoned and more frightened, which fills me with remorse and regret.

Katie: How it got noticed

At primary school I always had a few friends who I could almost hide behind. They took me under their wing so I was seen as shy but it didn't become too noticeable until my family moved and I started a new school. Being the new girl when everyone knew each other was difficult and I soon stood out.

It was at this school that the head-teacher noticed something was wrong and spoke to my parents about it. It was at this time, when I was ten years old, that the label 'Selective Mutism' was mentioned. My head-teacher said to my Mum, 'I don't want to scare you but she has difficulty speaking in class and I think it might be Selective Mutism. I would suggest that you go and see your doctor.'

After seeing the doctor, I was referred to a psychologist from the Community Health Team. Nothing was ever said to me, but judging by the way they dealt with me, I had the feeling people suspected that I had suffered some kind of trauma which had led me to stop talking. I remember having to take the morning off school to go to see the psychologist every week and it just felt like they were trying to get some kind of secret out of me as to why I wasn't speaking. I think back then SM wasn't ever heard of so people didn't understand it as much as they maybe would today. In my experience, it wouldn't surprise me if parents could be almost too scared to get proper help as it could look suspicious that their children seemed too scared to speak.

In the end I think the specialist nurse said, 'It's just her personality' and they decided to let it rest. When I went to secondary school they were told everything but just kept the information on file and didn't really do anything. It was in Year 8 when a teacher rang up my Mum and asked her what she thought about seeing a speech therapist. The speech therapist confirmed I had SM so I finally received an explanation about what was wrong with me. My Mum started to do some research and came across SMIRA.

It was a huge relief to finally understand the problem and to know that it was something I suffered from, not something that was wrong with me. Hearing other people's stories, I didn't feel so alone, and hearing how people had 'got over it' and lived normal lives made me feel like there was light at the end of the tunnel and things would get better. It felt like a community that it felt good to belong to.

Mother speaks: By the time Katie was ten the problem became more pronounced. I had thought about going to a psychologist but was again very wary that it would be misunderstood as a response to trauma or abuse. A speech therapist didn't seem appropriate as her speech was very well developed for her age. Eventually I did go to the family doctor but, as I feared, the CAMHS nurse didn't understand it either. In desperation I took her to various alternative health practitioners to no avail. The eventual diagnosis was a relief and SMIRA was a lifeline.

Katie: Bad experiences

Growing up, I remember hearing the phrase 'your school days are the best days of your life' and just thinking 'WHAT?!' Many people have fond memories of their school days and can reminisce with their school friends about all the fun they had, but this is something that I just can't relate to. My school days were in fact the worst days of my life.

Every day was filled with dread, loneliness and panic. I remember being too scared to sleep, as I knew what was waiting for me when I woke up. I would sometimes set my alarm for three hours before I actually needed to wake up just so I had time to mentally prepare myself for the day ahead.

Nobody ever wanted to be paired up with me in class and I was always last to be picked for everything. For example, if there were three of us in the group someone would say 'but there are only two of us, because we have Katie', as if I didn't count as a person.

Unsympathetic teachers made it even more difficult. I remember listening to a teacher praising a student after being paired with me (who was horrible to me and kicked up a fuss because she had to work with me), saying she knew how hard it was for someone to have to work with 'someone like that' (meaning me, as if I was being difficult). A PE teacher even shouted at me in front of the entire class, telling me I was 'letting everyone down'.

Teachers would say things like 'I know you don't like speaking but…' as if I had an attitude problem and was doing it on purpose. I found that really insulting and upsetting as I tried every day to speak normally but just couldn't. To me, it was like telling someone with hearing problems that they don't like to listen or someone with sight problems that they just weren't really looking.

I always had to look out for myself because people would treat me how they wanted because they knew I wouldn't tell anyone or fight back.

Naturally I struggled with oral exams in language subjects. Once at school I had revved myself up for ages in preparation for a speaking assessment in German, only to not be called in to the exam. It was assumed that I would not be taking part, even though I had done all the work and preparation as nobody had told me I wouldn't be doing the exam. It annoyed me that I was just ignored and pushed to one side and it was frustrating as I knew I was as capable as anyone else. I think in larger schools it is easy to just focus on a few people – the clever ones or the ones who cause trouble. The ones in between who don't cause any trouble are sometimes forgotten. In my last school I was supported a little bit more as my teacher recognized that I was perfectly able in other areas. However, when it came to my GCSEs I was excused from the oral assessments in English and German as it would have brought my final grade down unfairly. This time, however, I was actually informed that I would not be taking part and it was my choice rather than a decision that had been made for me.

When I was younger, the hardest part of all was that I didn't know what was wrong with me – nobody understood, not even myself – and I couldn't work out how to fix it. I was just stuck. I felt like the only person in the world that had this problem, which made it more isolating and lonely. In some ways I envied other people's problems as they could talk to other people about their issues. Nobody seemed to be able to empathize with me.

I spent most of my time at school by myself, being ignored by most people or having someone talk to me just because they were told to, when I could tell that they didn't want to.

Altogether I attended five different schools before I went to college. Every time I started a new school I always told myself 'this time it will be different' and 'when I make a fresh start I will start speaking and be normal and make friends'. But it never got any easier.

Katie: Different techniques used

Throughout my childhood it felt like I had tried everything possible to 'cure' my SM. I was taken to a homeopath, a cranial osteopath and a child hypnotherapist. I took medication such as Prozac and was offered bribes and rewards. The students at school were even given presentations about my problem in an attempt to help them understand and encourage them to include me and support me. But nothing really seemed to work.

Mother speaks: It was always rather obvious that as it was school where Katie was unable to speak it was in that environment that help should be given. Unfortunately, this never really happened. There was a limit to what we could do at home.

I remember when Katie was learning to swim; no amount of encouragement, pressure or rewards enabled her to find her confidence in the water. One day when we were in the pool with her brother and sisters and I left her to splash around I caught her out of the corner of my eye swimming a very elegant front crawl, completing almost a length of the pool. I always knew that Katie would be okay and would develop her social confidence as she had done in the water. Development should not be treated as a race. Looking back, I think it is about finding a balance between pressure and encouragement, not panicking but not giving up either. I remain full of regret that I was unable to find the appropriate resources to help her or help her myself when she was younger.

No one would know if they met Katie now what she has suffered. I know people are drawn to her quiet confidence. She is trustworthy, loyal, genuine, compassionate and has many and varied interests. Although her confidence can be knocked quite easily, she has developed a resilience and confidence that many would envy. Essentially, Katie confronted and resolved her problem through her own determination. However, involvement with SMIRA was the turning point and we are very grateful to everyone involved for their help and support.

Katie: *The cure*

I think in a way I knew that while I was at school I would never be able to talk normally and be part of the group. I did feel like everything would be so much easier once I left and that my life would start, so I used my time at school to get the best grades I could and as much experience as I could.

Sure enough, when I started college I began speaking to people. On my first day I was lucky enough to start speaking to someone who quickly became one of my best friends. As she was so chatty, confident and easy to talk to, she made friends quickly and her friends became my friends. Although I was still shy, lacked confidence and found it hard to speak up in classes, I found myself gaining more confidence and making more friends as time went on. Unlike school, I felt no pressure to start talking, it was just expected that I was normal and spoke to people and nobody made a big deal out of it when I did.

There were a couple of people at college who knew me from school and I was scared they would tell people how I used to be, which would prevent me from talking. I remember this happening at secondary school – I was speaking to someone in the first few days (or trying to) and the girl on the other side just turned round and said 'she doesn't talk' and the other girl kind of gave me a funny look and thought I was weird. Sure enough, I couldn't seem to talk to her.

University was the same, I started off a little shy and apprehensive but I grew in confidence and went on to join lots of groups and societies and even did a bit of public speaking, which made me feel quite proud.

Katie: The present

Looking back, I spent the first 18 years of my life in silence and isolation, suffering from something that made my life extremely difficult in a lot of ways. However, I now see this as my past and not something that will define me or affect my future. Because this is something that I suffered from when growing up, it is hard to tell what my life would be like if I didn't have it.

I try to stay positive and think about what I've gained from struggling with SM. As I missed out on the social side of school, I was determined to do well academically. I focused a lot of my energy and creativity into art and some people recognized my talent, which boosted my confidence a little. Because of my past experiences I think I have gained a lot of compassion and sensitivity towards other people.

I think it's made me more grateful for normal little things other people take for granted. I remember my first few weeks of college, talking and laughing with my new friends, just feeling so happy and so lucky to finally fit in.

I think there is a part of me that will always be a little bit shy and lack confidence in certain situations, but I know that this is okay and this is 'normal'. Most people suffer with confidence at some point in their lives, and if not, they are suffering with something else.

I want anyone else suffering from the same thing to know that things will be okay, no matter how long it goes on for and no matter how impossible it seems to be to ever be 'normal'.

Mina's story

Alice and Mina (not her real name) tell the story of how SMIRA and peers at school helped her recovery from SM.

Fourteen-year-old Mina appealed in writing to a mentor who was luckily employed at her secondary school. She had been performing well in all school subjects where speech was not needed but was not able to talk to teachers or peers. She really wanted to overcome her problem and was brave enough to make the first approach. The mentor had heard of SMIRA and contacted the charity for advice. It was clear that Mina was suffering from SM and could be helped.

Mina's father explained that his daughter could talk to most, though not quite all, of their extended family at home, so it seemed that a 'Circle of Friends' approach (Taylor 1997) might well succeed, especially if personal contact was maintained with SMIRA through Alice Sluckin.

With encouragement from the school in the shape of drinks and biscuits, a support group was set up and several girls from Mina's class volunteered to join. Alice and the school mentor were also members of the group. Meetings were only held once a month and Mina still did not talk, but mutual disclosure of how they felt about being at school and why certain topics interested them seemed to bring the girls closer. Mina was no longer isolated at break times and began to look much happier. Mina was able to hold lively 'conversations' with Alice by means of writing her replies and remained in regular contact.

Then careful thought was given to the question of 'work experience' and the school staff were able to arrange placement at a nursery. After a few weeks Mina began to talk to the nursery children and then the staff. It was during this period that she also began speaking to Alice and the school mentor.

The compulsory oral elements of public exams in both English and French were the next big hurdles, but the school came up with the idea that it would be helpful for the 'circle of friends' to be present in the exam room. This was allowed and Mina spoke audibly and passed.

This was a successful but slow programme of support and hard work for all concerned. It had taken two and a half years to get from silence to confident speech. However, the value can be seen in the fact that transfer to Sixth Form College went smoothly and Mina then progressed to university where she is now studying her chosen subject.

It is a measure of the school's involvement and understanding that a decision was taken to award Mina a special prize for having overcome her fear of talking.

The story from Mina's point of view in her own words

It's been five years since I fully overcame SM. I am now 21 and currently doing a university degree. I am happy, talkative and my confidence has increased throughout the years. It all started back in nursery. I don't know exactly how it started. Was it because someone had said something to me? It all remains a mystery.

At home, I was like any other child – laughing, playing with my toys, watching kids' programmes and talking to my family – but at nursery, I was a completely different person. I wasn't able to socialize, talk, laugh. I was constantly anxious, and my face and body language were expressionless. This was due to my social anxiety disorder SM. It was not because I didn't want to talk. I really did want to talk and make friends, smile and laugh, but anxiety took over, which prevented me from being myself. I was not only anxious at nursery, but outside my home wherever I went, such as shops or my cousins' houses. The list can go on.

I felt like an alien whenever I walked into a classroom. There was always someone who would either say something about me or whisper something about me during class. Some people would even come up to me and ask why I didn't talk. It made me feel anxious and I hated myself when people came up to me and asked why I didn't talk. I felt anxious and self-conscious and I hated myself for it. I hated the fact that I was afraid to speak. I hated the fact that I was unable to stand up for myself. Most nights I went to bed crying because it seemed as if SM was taking over my life. Even talking to my grandmother and some of my aunties and uncles was impossible.

The three words that irritated me the most were 'She can't talk'. I used to hear this almost every day at school. I wanted to say 'I can talk', but unfortunately I was unable to due to my severe anxiety. I used to ask myself every day, 'Why me?' 'Why does this happen to me?' I blamed myself because it was my fault that I didn't talk. It was my fault that I was getting bullied. Everything was my fault. But now looking back, I realize it wasn't my fault as I couldn't help the way I was. In an unusual way, I'm glad I had SM, as it has transformed me into a wiser person and it has made me believe that nothing is impossible if you put your mind into it. It has also taught me to never judge someone, as you don't know what happens behind closed doors.

My friends and family, especially my father, supported me and understood my anxiety. There was also the SMIRA counsellor, Alice, who helped me overcome my anxiety. She was very helpful and gave great advice and techniques. The technique that helped me most was setting realistic targets from easiest to hardest. It was like stepping up a ladder every time I accomplished each target, the ladder to success (Figure 16.1).

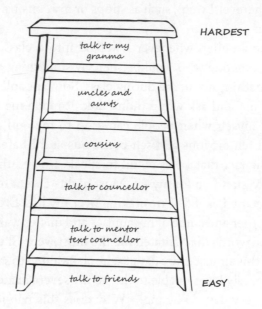

HARDEST

talk to my
granma

uncles and
aunts

cousins

talk to councellor

talk to mentor
text councellor

talk to friends   EASY

Figure 16.1 The ladder to success

Also, knowing that there were other people out there with SM made me feel less of an alien. I was not the only person in the world with this disorder. Reading inspirational stories about others overcoming SM motivated me into overcoming my anxiety. Even though not everyone believed that I would overcome it, I had faith in myself that I would, no matter how long it would take. In contrast to my outer appearance – timid, anxious and shy – there was strength, faith and motivation on the inside.

Advice I would give to people who suffer from SM is: never give up, because you will overcome it, however long it takes. It can take months, or even years, but you WILL overcome it.

Remind yourself that you are not the only one going through this, and that, when you accomplish each target – no matter how small – it is a step closer to success. Believe in yourself, have faith and, though this may be easier said than done, try your best not to let other people's comments bring you down. If they have a problem, it's theirs, not yours. You are you and if anyone decides to judge you then they are not worthy of your time.

Don't ever lose hope. You can beat SM.

CHAPTER 17

Summary and Recommendations for the Future

Alice Sluckin and Rae Smith

What has been learnt from the contributors?

We have seen in this volume that attitudes and beliefs around children who fail to speak in specific situations have changed over the decades. These children do not form a homogeneous group. The term 'Selective Mutism' (SM) identifies their behaviour rather than their disorder. Viana *et al.* (2009) felt that a developmental psychopathology perspective, contrary to an 'either/or' view, might be particularly helpful when considering the complexities of SM (p.65). However, it is now known that the great majority of these silent children suffer from an anxiety disorder and can also have additional problems which require attention (Yeganeh *et al.* 2003). Parents have presented us with new information about their SM children and we have also heard from some of the children themselves. We have seen that concerns about children affected by SM are leading parents and professionals to set up effective support groups, both here in the UK and abroad.

Diagnosis of SM has sometimes been complicated by 'exclusions'. Whether it is helpful to say that a child with an additional diagnosis should not be described as having SM may depend on local policies. We were pleased to be able to include chapters discussing 'co-morbidity' of SM with communication disorders and the autistic spectrum.

Another chapter described how medication may have helped a young man who is now free from SM, and a child psychiatrist discusses this topic further.

We were grateful to the local authority workers who explained how services offered in community settings helped individual children to begin, in some cases quite rapidly, to talk at school. A music therapist later showed how similarly rapid results can be obtained. We would like to stress, however, that quick cures are not necessarily permanent. Some children need ongoing support to prevent relapse, especially at transition points – for instance, when they face a change of school or teacher.

In another chapter, parents, children and young people described how, with the support of SMIRA, they overcame SM very gradually, step by difficult step – in some cases permanently.

Details of the administrative arrangements for providing services for SM and the legal framework that supports these services in the UK were provided. Also, for comparison, we included descriptions of the SM situation in some other countries.

The vital related issue of confidence was discussed, towards the end of the book, by a specialist who has been providing classes to promote this for children and adolescents in schools and colleges over many years with excellent results.

The recovery of two young adults by means of personal determination, consultation with SMIRA and the establishment of friendships within the peer group was described. In contrast to these achievements, a valuable appendix (see page 272) describes a research project exploring the situation and views of adults, many of whom were not helped as children and did not have the same opportunity to put the problem of SM behind them.

In this final chapter we suggest some possible future developments. Key messages from the previous chapters have been that many SM children long to communicate and will respond to sympathetic (but not overindulgent) guidance. We know what type of help is available and we know that it should be offered at the earliest possible stage, so that SM children's anxiety does not go on to become a lifetime burden.

Understanding anxiety

A significant contribution to the understanding of anxiety and SM has been made by Rachel Klein, Professor of Clinical Psychology, University of New York Child Study Centre. She had been a member of the Review Committee which was set up during the preparation of *DSM-IV* which was the previous version of *DSM-5* mentioned throughout this book.

The committee's recommendation at that time was that the disorder previously known as 'Elective Mutism' be renamed 'Selective Mutism' since no evidence was found that situationally silent children had a deliberate preference not to speak (personal communication 1992). It was also noted that the majority were very anxious.

Professor Klein is the author of a most informative paper (Klein 2009) introducing the classification of anxiety disorders current at that time.

It may be helpful to clarify the meaning of 'anxiety', which is an emotional state maintained in anticipation and preparation for future imagined events. An anxiety state is complicated by many factors, some internal and others external. It is related to 'fear', which is a simpler, more direct response to current danger, preparing the body for fight or flight.

SM is now much more widely acknowledged to be an anxiety condition and many speech and language therapists and teachers have understood that some SM children may be making unconscious use of what is known as a 'safety behaviour' to deal with overwhelming anxiety. Confusingly, careful observation of an SM child may lead one to the false conclusion that s/he is simply choosing not to speak and is not feeling at all anxious. This observation can lead to impatience and criticism when the crucial piece of information previously mentioned in our introduction and in Chapter 15 is missing, that is, by avoiding verbal interaction in anxiety-provoking situations, children can feel relatively comfortable. They have successfully sidestepped their worries. People who fear they may stammer sometimes achieve a similar result by means of 'avoidance' – for instance, by keeping utterances short or substituting safer choices for difficult words thus concealing their difficulty.

Sweeney *et al.* (2013, p.90) state: 'Avoidance is anxiety's best friend. Avoiding feared situations permits the anxiety to further develop and become more fully integrated into one's life. The skills taught in psychosocial treatments are in service of facilitating the individual's engagement of the feared situation in order to neutralize and extinguish the fear.'

Is there a genetic explanation?

There is now general agreement that SM may be related to social phobias and that there is often a family history of shyness, or avoidance.

In 2007 an internet questionnaire was given through SMIRA to parents of SM children, and 53 members replied. Thirty-eight were parents of girls and 15 of boys. Forty-seven individual parents reported a history of family shyness. This ratio confirms literature reports (Cline and Baldwin 2004; Roe 2011). However, it is thought to be an oversimplification to ascribe complex behaviour patterns purely to genetic factors. The environment and family lifestyle that children are exposed to from the very beginning is known to exert a major influence. Also, the child's inborn temperament will play a part. As mentioned in Chapter 10, some children show 'behavioural inhibition to the unfamiliar' (Kagan and Snidman 2004). It was found that this applied to 10–15 per cent of newborns.

A recent paper describing parenting interventions for young anxious children (Laskey 2011) stresses the need to investigate how parents manage stressful interactions and also how they react to their children's anxiety. Laskey's view is that both overly rigid and overly lax parenting have the potential to increase a child's vulnerability to anxiety. A rigid upbringing can undermine a child's autonomy and confidence to try new experiences, while lax parenting can deprive children of the supportive structure which is needed to discourage avoidance.

It also seems possible that anxious mothers have a tendency to overprotect their children. Aktar *et al.* (2014) found that the babies of mothers with lifetime diagnoses of Social Anxiety Disorder (SAD) became progressively more afraid of strangers. At 30 months they showed higher levels of fear and avoidance than the children of mothers without this diagnosis.

The findings in Aktar's research were specific to SAD, but there could also be an association with SM. Families might therefore like to consider seeking help for their own discomfort, not just that of their child.

Where should help be offered?

Another concern of Rachel Klein's was that children with anxiety disorders were not being referred. At that time, she noted: 'The majority of children with anxiety disorders are not referred for treatment. To enable identification and treatment of children with anxiety intervention will need to be implemented in non-psychiatric settings such as schools and Primary Health Care settings' (Klein 2009, p.158).

Up to a point, this is also the position of the editors with regard to SM. Schools will often be the places where effective, long-term help can best be organized and parents supported, though schools may not always be fully prepared for this responsibility.

Since 2007, schools in the UK have had a duty to foster their pupils' mental health as well as their academic development. A succession of government initiatives have sought to include emotional health and development in educational objectives. One such initiative is the Targeted Mental Health in Schools Project (2008).

However, when Vostanis *et al.* (2013) conducted a baseline study looking at schools' capacity to undertake this additional duty, shortcomings were found. Five hundred and ninety-nine primary schools and 137 secondary schools were approached and it was found that, although two-thirds of the schools did focus on all aspects of the children's mental health, they concentrated on reactive rather than preventive interventions. Support for teachers in this new role in the form of consultation, counselling and training was limited. The editorial of the publication in which the Vostanis study appeared (Weare 2013) is forthright in pointing to the central importance of adopting preventative approaches, which necessitate improvements in staff support, morale and preparation.

Unfortunately, anxious children in need of help are often seen by organizations isolated from one another and there is at present little co-ordination, joint funding or information-sharing between schools, Social Services, Community Health and CAMHS. This may particularly apply to very young children who are at the stage where intervention is likely to be most successful.

Despite this, we suggest that a fruitful approach for SM might be the greater involvement of CAMHS teams. An advantage of this could be that Cognitive Behavioural Therapy (CBT) would become more readily available.

What types of intervention can be recommended?

Commenting on prevention and treatment, Klein (2009) stated that substantial progress had already been made by using systems such as CBT, possibly combined with medication. CBT aims to change children's anxious thinking and also the thinking of their anxious parents. It also aims to reduce their fearfulness by encouraging them to alter their behaviour by very small steps. Where SM is concerned, the therapist or helper needs to understand in considerable detail just how complex successful communicative behaviour actually is, so as to be able to break it down into sufficiently small units. The absence of these minute graduations of difficulty may explain why CBT, given alone, has not to date recorded great success with improving the actual communication of SM people, although their anxious thinking may well have been brought under control. Another factor may be that the therapists have found it difficult to deal with non-speaking patients.

Speech and Language Therapists (SLTs) are often able to provide the detailed breakdown that is needed (see Johnson and Wintgens 2001 and also Katz-Bernstein in Chapter 12 of this volume) while parents, teachers and learning support assistants are in an excellent position to put it into practice day by day (see Chapters 9 and 10 of this volume and also Robinson and Burges 2001).

It is relevant that Law and Garrett (2004) suggested that, in view of the relationship in childhood between speech–language–communication and behavioural difficulties: 'There is clearly a case for integration of the provision to these children and this should be reflected in clinical guidelines and good practice recommendations' (p.54). A strong emphasis on co-operative preventive SLT policies can also be found in Law, Reilly and Snow (2013).

As people who often gain detailed knowledge of the 'small steps' approach to restoring actual speech, parents can play a vital role in delivering more effective, holistic CBT to SM children. Studies in the past have shown that there may be a significant reduction in children's anxiety when intervention is delivered by their parents, guided by therapists. A recent randomized control trial undertaken by a group of clinical psychologists (Thirlwall *et al.* 2013) involving 194 children found that parents who were supported and guided to use a self-help book (Creswell and Willetts 2007) and CBT to reduce their children's anxiety achieved excellent results. In this particular study the parents did not themselves have diagnosed anxiety disorders. We need to acknowledge that parents who are themselves anxious will find it understandably harder to encourage their timid children to face life's challenges. Murray *et al.* (2008), for example, found that, unfortunately, anxious mothers tended to encourage avoidance in anxious children, thereby increasing their vulnerability. Consistent and ongoing support and encouragement for the whole family may be the key. A very useful handbook *From Timid to Tiger* has been produced by Cartwright-Hatton *et al.* (2010) for professionals aiming to support anxious parents. The light-hearted, yet sympathetic, tone of this book makes it particularly suitable for helping families where a timid and avoidant approach to life has become an unintentional habit.

Avoiding negative adult input

We have seen that teachers and nursery staff are viewed as crucial by people who have suffered from SM. Stories of their struggle with the condition often focus on terrifying experiences with these powerful adults or on lifelong gratitude to heroic rescuers from among the same group. The adults in our Appendix also describe teachers as having been important.

The little girl whose fictional account of SM (Johnson and Wintgens 2012) inspired us to begin this book devotes nine pages to teachers and asks them, above all, to be understanding. Unfortunately, this is not always easy. Few confident people can imagine what it feels like to be unable to respond when expected to talk. On the other hand, most of us fully sympathize with the feelings of hurt, frustration and impotence experienced by the person on the other end of the silence. Therein lies a problem for situationally mute people; they are frequently criticized but seldom understood. Indeed, even the professional view of their silence was at one time highly critical. We have seen that they were labelled 'Elective Mutes' and were widely perceived as 'speech refusers', manipulative, rejecting, controlling and hostile. Unsurprisingly, their condition was then regarded as intractable, since indignant demands for speech serve only to increase situational anxiety.

The fact that we now know better does not always bring our hurt feelings under control when children appear rudely silent, though it should.

What should now be done to improve the lives of children and families where someone is selectively mute?

- Diagnostic exclusions which prevent SM children from accessing services should be ignored. Professor Sir Michael Rutter (2008, p.211) stated in the context of language disorders, diagnostic concepts and risk processes: 'Fortunately, in the United Kingdom most services do not operate in a "tick box" diagnostic fashion… On the other hand, some services unfortunately do have a tick-box approach, and for them it is reasonable to use the label that provides an entry ticket.' We take this to mean that common sense should be applied.

- The availability of information about SM should be improved. Reaching the relevant professional groups as well as parents and carers is essential. National guidelines, similar to those available in relation to autism, would improve the identification, handling and remediation of SM.

- The National Institute for Health and Care Excellence (NICE) has been asked to consider recommending early assessment and intervention for SM children in order to safeguard their mental health.

- The evidence base concerning management and remediation of SM needs to be strengthened. Experience has shown that several types of intervention for SM can be successful and several studies in the past supported this. Recently, a randomized controlled trial conducted in Norway (Oerbeck *et al.* 2013) confirmed that good progress can be expected, especially if help is offered at an early age. We would add 'or at a time of emotional readiness'. However, the evidence base still needs to be strengthened. The need for follow-up and ongoing support also requires investigation. As shown in Chapters 9 and 12, children who have suffered from SM are apt to experience any major life-change as challenging.

- Researchers may like to consider projects concerning the efficacy and cost-effectiveness of the following approaches:

  o Affordable, 'ice-breaking' interventions such as those described by Roe (1993, 2004) and in Chapter 9 of this volume

  o Parent-assisted, step-by-step behavioural treatment as described in Chapter 10

  o Combinations of either of these with CBT therapies

- ○   Pet/animal support for SM children

- ○   All types of music therapy for SM

- ○   Intervention strategies for SM in adults.

Further research questions

- • What is the true incidence of SM? We suspect that it is more prevalent than was previously thought, as do Sharkey and McNicholas (2012). These child psychiatrists share Klein's impression, referred to above, that not all SM children are referred for treatment, but also identify some of the factors that make it difficult to gain reliable information about the incidence of this disorder.

- • Are there selectively mute children without recognized anxiety disorder? If so, what may account for their silence and what kind of help do they need?

- • Does recognition of sub-groups within SM yield more reliable information than treating it as a unitary phenomenon?

Our primary recommendation

The development of a young child's situational silence into a costly and harmful long-term condition appears to be most easily avoidable if it is tackled early. However, in Chapter 2 of this book Tony Cline points out that 'There are no published data on the incidence of SM in nurseries and playgroups. Relatively few referrals are recorded' (from those settings).

We would therefore like to see all health visitors, social workers and nursery staff receive basic training in the recognition and initial management of SM in young children, with special attention being given to appropriate parent guidance and support. Some primary school and nursery staff should receive more advanced training in remedial approaches to SM.

GPs, paediatricians and service commissioners, psychiatrists and psychologists need access to reliable information about SM, as do families and the wider children's work force.

Commissioners in particular will then be in a position to embark on preventive joint commissioning (health/education/social care) in one of the areas of child mental health as recommended by the campaign group Young Minds (Brennan 2013).

Together with parents, the people identified above can ensure that environments are adapted so as to be less overwhelming to the anxious child. In a nutshell: the demand for speech must be discontinued and non-verbal communication and noisy play, within and beyond the home, must be encouraged. Facilitation groups such as that described by Roe (1993, 2004) also have a part to play. Having said this, we hope to have shown that some children – for example, Ann in Chapter 10 and the two formerly SM adults in Chapter 16 – need time to mature before their SM can be overcome and that success can be achieved at later stages, given the requisite information, motivation and support.

We hope the book will help to release some previously unheard voices.

Selective Mutism in Adults

Carl Sutton

iSpeak is a non-profit organization which I formed in early 2012: (a) to address the lack of professional understanding and support for older teenagers and adults with Selective Mutism (SM); (b) to counter the popular perception that SM is 'just' a childhood disorder; and (c) to provide a sufferer-led view of SM. We provide primarily online support for older teenagers and adults with SM, support to parents, advice to practitioners, and conduct academic research on SM.

Throughout 2013, during a Psychology conversion MSc at the University of Chester (UK), I conducted the first study of SM in adults. The study was advertised online on the iSpeak website, the SMG~CAN website, and through word-of-mouth by SMIRA.

It was demonstrated that a significant number of adults continue to experience SM; that is to say they speak freely in some situations but feel themselves consistently unable to talk in others. Eighty-three adults from 11 countries took part in the study, responding online or via paper questionnaires, the majority coming from the UK and USA. All participants indicated that they experienced SM beyond age 18. Seventy-nine adults said they were still suffering with SM at the time of taking part in the study. The age range of participants was between 18 and 64, with a mean age of 33.4. In agreement with all other studies on SM, which indicate that the onset of the disorder is generally between two and four years of age, the mean age of onset for adults with SM in this sample was 3.78.

There was a much higher gender ratio than in any other study on SM – of approximately four females to one male. Some of this bias may be due to adult males being more likely to self-stigmatize and thus being less likely to take part in this kind of research; however, it does cast some doubt on the 1:1 gender ratio indicated in *DSM-5* (APA 2013), particularly when one considers that all other anxiety disorders (which *DSM-5* now categorizes SM as) have a female preponderance of between 2:1 and 3:1.

Interestingly, seven of the adults with SM who took part (all mothers) had children with SM – indicating a genetic, predisposing and/or social-learning aspect to SM. Additionally, the majority of respondents suggested that the trigger for their SM had been minor or there had been no memorable trigger at all. However, 22 per cent indicated that abuse in the childhood home (emotional, physical and/or vicarious – e.g. witnessing domestic violence) had triggered or compounded their SM; and 40 per cent indicated that bullying at school had triggered or compounded their SM. SM is thus likely to be a gene plus environment interaction, occurring for multifarious reasons, including no reason, and including (infrequently) stressors at home.

The study addressed a number of key questions relating to the long-term course of the disorder and adult co-morbidities for the estimated 23 per cent of children with SM whose SM continues into adulthood.

First of all the study clearly demonstrated that SM in adults exists; a simple 'finding' which needs to be stated because the majority of academic research is on children with SM and further that SM in adults is uncommon, but not rare. While mean peak severity of the disorder appears to occur between ages 12 and 19, severity generally decreasing thereafter until around age 60, some adults (particularly those who reported significant stressors in childhood) continue to experience SM into their 50s.

Many adults with SM lead fulfilled lives, have life partners, and, in many cases, work. This is not to say it is easy, however, as many express the difficulties they have progressing at work. Among adults with a degree of SM there are teachers, lecturers, artists, people in caring and medical professions and (in my own case) a software engineer. On the other hand, there are also many adults with SM who can barely leave the house alone, experiencing agoraphobia in addition to SM and are thus unable to seek employment – interviews being the first major hurdle. This would suggest that access to benefits may also be a problem for them.

Second, the research also showed that only around 25 per cent of adults with SM received diagnoses of SM in childhood; a further 25 per cent of adults with SM indicated that, as children, their parents were unaware of their SM; and a further 25 per cent of adults with SM had parents who were aware of their child's difference but did not know SM was a known condition per se and did not seek help for their children.

Things appear to be 'improving' in this regard, however. Younger participants were more likely to have received a diagnosis, which may indicate that diagnosis rates have increased, particularly post-1994 (after publication of *DSM-IV*, the beginning of the influence of organizations such as SMIRA, and at the beginning of the rapid growth of the internet).

Interestingly, the diagnosis rates in the UK and USA appear to be roughly the same. However, it should also be noted that diagnosis in childhood does not predict recovery by adulthood, according to this study. A diagnosis in itself is worthless without appropriate and effective therapeutic intervention. Those taking part in this study who received diagnoses as children became adults with SM, even if they received treatment as children. In fact, many adults with SM cited the intervention they received as unhelpful or detrimental, though the types of treatment offered are unfortunately not known. At this juncture, professional awareness of SM in adults appears to be poor/non-existent and there is nowhere for adults with SM to turn.

Third, according to this research, adults with SM are very significantly more likely than the general population to develop other mood- and anxiety-related conditions, most notably depression, anxiety, panic disorder, social anxiety and PTSD. For some, chronic mental health conditions are a factor in their lives. Most indicated that they felt their long-term mental health conditions could have been avoided with appropriate support at the appropriate time in childhood. Adults with SM indicated what could have helped most was: (a) better understanding of SM in the school system; (b) access to counselling or CBT in childhood; and/or (c) access to speech therapy services. Of professionals, with exceptions (some teachers having been helpful), teachers were noted to be both the least likely to help with SM and most likely to make SM worse.

This study focused on the relationship between social anxiety and SM, and indicated that social anxiety was an almost universal co-morbidity by age 12. In fact, for the majority (72%) SM appeared to develop as a result of precocious social anxiety. For this group, SM may be a specific manifestation of SAD. For the remainder (28%), social anxiety appeared to develop as a result of having SM – that is, they became socially anxious because they found themselves unable to speak in certain circumstances, rather than because they were socially anxious per se. As such, the research suggests that for some (particularly for those who are younger than age 12) SM and SAD are differentiable and, thus, that the APA made the correct decision in *DSM-5* to keep SM and SAD separate. By way of example, it would be difficult to argue that mutism which occurs in the home environment with parents (as it did for some participants in this study – and as it did for me) is, itself, simply 'social' anxiety.

For more information on this study, contact carl@ispeak.org.uk.

References

Adams, C. (2005) 'Social communication intervention for school-age children: rationale and description.' *Seminars in Speech and Language 26*, 3, 181–188.

Adams, C. (2008) 'Intervention for Children with Pragmatic Language Impairments.' In C.F. Norbury, J.B. Tomblin and D.V.M. Bishop (eds) *Understanding Developmental Language Disorders. From Theory to Practice.* New York, NY: Psychology Press.

Aktar, E., Majdandžić, M., de Vente, W. and Bögels, M. (2014) 'Parental social anxiety disorder prospectively predicts toddlers' fear/avoidance in a social referencing paradigm.' *Journal of Child Psychology and Psychiatry 55*, 1, 77–87.

American Psychiatric Association (1994) *Diagnostic and Statistical Manual of Mental Disorders (4th edition).* Washington, DC: American Psychiatric Publishing.

American Psychiatric Association (2013) *Diagnostic and Statistical Manual of Mental Disorders (5th edition).* Washington, DC: American Psychiatric Publishing.

Amir, D. (2005) 'Re-finding the voice: music therapy with a girl who has selective mutism.' *Nordic Journal of Music Therapy 14*, 1, 67–78.

Anstendig, K. (1998) 'Selective mutism: a review of the treatment literature by modality from 1980–1996.' *Psychotherapy: Theory, Research, Practice, Training 35*, 3, 381–391.

Anstendig, K. (1999) 'Is selective mutism an anxiety disorder? Rethinking its DSM-IV classification.' *Journal of Anxiety Disorders 13*, 4, 417–434.

Baron-Cohen, S. (2003) *The Essential Difference.* London: Penguin.

Beck, J.S. (1995) *Cognitive Therapy: Basics and Beyond.* New York, NY: The Guilford Press.

Beer, J., Lombardo, M. and Bhanji, J. (2010) 'Roles of medial prefrontal cortex and orbitofrontal cortex in self-evaluation.' *Journal of Cognitive Neuroscience 22*, 9, 2108–2119.

Bercow, J. (2008) *Review of Services for Children and Young People (0–19) with Speech, Language and Communication Needs.* London: HMSO.

Bergman, R.L. (2013) *Treatment for Children with Selective Mutism: An Integrative Behavioural Approach.* Oxford: Oxford University Press.

Bergman, R., Keller, M., Piacentini, J. and Bergman, A. (2008) 'The development and psychometric properties of the Selective Mutism Questionnaire.' *Journal of Clinical Child and Adolescent Psychology 37*, 456–464.

Bergman, R.L., Piacentini, J. and McCracken, J.T. (2002) 'Prevalence and description of Selective Mutism in a school-based sample.' *Journal of the American Academy of Child and Adolescent Psychiatry 41*, 8, 9038–9046.

Bishop, D.V.M. (2008) 'Specific Language Impairment, Dyslexia, and Autism: Using Genetics to Unravel their Relationship.' In C.F. Norbury, J.B. Tomblin and D.V.M. Bishop (eds) *Understanding Developmental Language Disorders. From Theory to Practice.* New York, NY: Psychology Press.

Black, B. and Uhde, T.W. (1992) 'Elective mutism as a variant of social phobia.' *Journal of the American Academy of Child and Adolescent Psychiatry 31*, 6, 1090–1094.

Black, B. and Uhde, T.W. (1994) 'Treatment of elective mutism with fluoxetine: a double-blind , placebo-controlled study.' *Journal of the American Academy of Child and Adolescent Psychiatry 33*, 7, 1000–1006.

Black, B. and Uhde, T.W. (1995) 'Psychiatric characteristics of children with selective mutism: a pilot study.' *Journal of the American Academy of Child and Adolescent Psychiatry 34*, 7, 847–856.

Bloodstein, O. and Bernstein-Ratner, N. (2007) *A Handbook on Stuttering.* Clifton Park, NY: Thomson/Cengage.

Brennan, S. (2013) 'Two steps forward.' *Young Minds 122*, 19.

Brown, B. and Lloyd, H. (1975) 'A controlled study of children not speaking at school.' *Journal of the Association of Workers for Maladjusted Children 3*, 49–63.

Buck, M. (1988) 'The silent children.' *Special Children 22*, 12–15.

Carlson, J.S., Kratochwill, T.R. and Johnston, H.F. (1999) 'Sertraline treatment of 5 children diagnosed with selective mutism: a single-case research trial.' *Journal of Child and Adolescent Psychopharmacology 9*, 4, 293–230.

Carmody, L. (2000) 'The power of silence: selective mutism in Ireland – a speech and language perspective.' *Journal of Clinical Speech and Language Studies 1*, 41–60.

Cartwright-Hatton, S., Laskey, B., Rust, S. and McNally, D. (2010) *From Timid to Tiger: A Treatment Manual for Parenting the Anxious Child.* Chichester: Wiley.

Chandra, Y. (1999) *The Dictionary of Psychology.* New York, NY: Psychology Press.

Cleator, H.M. (1998) *Speech and Language Characteristics of Selectively Mute Children: A Speech Pathology Perspective.* Unpublished Master's Thesis, University of Sydney.

Cleator, H.M. and Hand, L.S. (2001) 'Selective mutism: how a successful speech and language assessment really is possible.' *International Journal of Language and Communication Disorders 36*, Supplement, 126–131.

Cline, T. and Baldwin, S. (2004) *Selective Mutism in Children.* London: Whurr. (First published 1995.)

Cohan, S.L., Chavira, D.A., Shipton-Blum, E., Hitchcock, C., Roesch, S.C. and Stein, M.B. (2008) 'Refining the classification of children with selective mutism: a latent profile analysis.' *Journal of Clinical Child and Adolescent Psychiatry 37*, 4, 770–784.

Cohan, S.L., Price, J.M. and Stein, M.B. (2006) 'Suffering in silence: why a developmental psychopathology perspective on selective mutism is needed.' *Journal of Developmental and Behavioural Paediatrics 27*, 4, 341–355.

Colligan, R.W., Colligan, R.C. and Dilliard, M.K. (1977) 'Contingency management in the classroom treatment of long-term elective mutism: a case report.' *Journal of School Psychology 15*, 1, 9–17.

Creswell, C., and Willetts, L. (2007) *Overcoming your Child's Fears and Worries: A Guide for Parents Using Cognitive Behavioural Techniques.* London: Robinson.

Crogan, L.M. and Craven, R. (1982) 'Elective mutism: learning from the analysis of a successful case history.' *Journal of Paediatric Psychology 7*, 1, 85–93.

Crystal, D. (1997) *The Cambridge Encyclopaedia of Language (2nd edition).* Cambridge: Cambridge University Press.

Cummings, L. (2009) *Clinical Pragmatics.* Cambridge: Cambridge University Press.

Cunningham, C.E., Cataldo, M.F., Mallion, C. and Keyes, J.B. (1983) 'Evaluation of behavioural approaches to the management of selective mutism.' *Child and Family Behaviour Therapy 5*, 4, 25–49.

Cunningham, C.E., McHolm, A., Boyle, M.H. and Patel, S. (2004) 'Behavioral and emotional adjustment, family functioning, academic performance, and social relationships in children with selective mutism.' *Journal of Child Psychology and Psychiatry 45*, 8, 1363–1372.

Danon-Boileau, L. (2001) *The Silent Child* (English translation). New York, NY: Oxford University Press. (First published 1995, Calmann-Levy.)

Darnley-Smith, R. and Patey, H.M. (2003) *Music Therapy.* Thousand Oaks, CA: Sage.

Davis, S. (2013) *Susie Has Selective Mutism.* Kirkby in Ashfield: Specialdirect.

Department for Children, Schools and Families (2008) *Targeted Mental Health in Schools Project.* Nottingham: DCSF.

Department for Education and Skills (2001) *Special Educational Needs Code of Practice – No. 58.* London: DfES.

Department for Education and Skills (2007) *Social and Emotional Aspects of Learning for Secondary Schools (SEAL): Guidance Booklet.* Nottingham: DfES.

Dillon, J. and Malony, A. (2013) *The Cat that Unlocked a Boy's Heart: Jessi-Cat.* London: Michael O'Mara.

Dow, S.P., Sonies, B.C., Scheib, D., Moss, S.E. and Leonard, H.L. (1995) 'Practical guidelines for the assessment and treatment of selective mutism.' *Journal of the American Academy of Child and Adolescent Psychiatry 24*, 7, 836–846.

Dow, S.P., Sonies, B.C., Scheib, C., Moss, S.E. and Leonard, H.L. (1999) 'Practical Guidelines for the Assessment and Treatment of Selective Mutism.' In S.A. Spasaro and C.E. Schaefer (eds) *Refusal to Speak. Treatment of Selective Mutism in Children.* Northvale, NJ: Jason Aronson.

Dowrick, P.W. (1983) 'Self-modelling.' In S.J. Biggs (ed.) *Using Video: Psychological and Social Applications.* Chichester: Wiley.

Dowrick, P.W. and Hood, M. (1978) 'Transfer of Talking Behaviours Across Settings Using Faked Films.' In E.L. Glynn and S.S. McNaughton (eds) *New Zealand Conference for Research in Applied Behavioural Analysis.* Auckland: Auckland University Press.

Duffy, J.R. (2005) *Motor Speech Disorders: Substrates, Differential Diagnosis and Management.* St. Louis, MO: Mosby.

Dummit, E.S., Klein, R.G., Tancer, N.K., Asche, B., Martin, J., and Fairbanks, J.A. (1997) 'Systematic assessment of 50 children with selective mutism.' *Journal of the American Academy of Child and Adolescent Psychiatry 36,* 5, 653–660.

Elizalde-Utnick, G. (2007) 'Young selectively mute English language learners: school based intervention strategies.' *Journal of Early Childhood and Infant Psychology 3,* 141–162.

Elizur, Y. and Perednik, R. (2003) 'Prevalence and description of selective mutism in immigrant and native families: a controlled study.' *Journal of the American Academy of Child and Adolescent Psychiatry 42,* 12, 1451–1459.

Elson, A., Pearson, C., Jones, C.D. and Schumacher, E. (1965) 'Followup study of childhood elective mutism.' *Archives of General Psychiatry 13,* 2, 182–187.

Engel, G.L. (1980) 'The clinical application of the biopsychosocial model.' *American Journal of Psychiatry 137,* 5, 535–545.

Erikson, E.H. (1963) *Childhood and Society.* New York, NY: Norton. (Originally published 1950.)

Ford, M.A., Sladeczek, I.E., Carlson, J. and Kratochwill, T.R. (1998) 'Selective mutism: phenomenological characteristics.' *School Psychology Quarterly 13,* 3, 192–227.

Gibbons, J. (1985) 'The silent period: an examination.' *Language Learning 35,* 2, 255–267.

Golwyn, H. and Weinstock, R.C. (1990) 'Phenelzine treatment of elective mutism: a case report.' *Journal of Clinical Psychiatry 51,* 9, 384–385.

Guitar, B. (2006) *Stuttering: An Integrated Approach to Its Nature and Treatment (3rd edition).* Philadelphia, PA: Lippincott Williams and Wilkins.

Hadley, N.H. (1994) *Elective Mutism: A Handbook for Educators, Counsellors and Health Care Practitioners.* Dordrecht: Kluwer.

Halpern, W.I., Hammond, J. and Cohen, R. (1971) 'A therapeutic approach to speech phobia: elective mutism reexamined.' *Journal of the American Academy of Child Psychiatry 10,* 1, 94–107.

Hall, A. (2008) 'Ready to talk...' *Times Educational Supplement/Selective Mutism Supplement*, 3 October 2008, p.6.

Harrison, L.J., McLeod, S., Berthelsen, D. and Walker, S. (2009) 'Literacy, numeracy, and learning in school-aged children identified as having speech and language impairment in early childhood.' *International Journal of Speech-Language Pathology 11*, 5, 392–403.

Hartman, B. (1997) *Mutismus: Zur Theorie und Kasuistik des Totalen und Elektiven Mutismus.* Berlin: Marhold.

Hartman, B. (2006) *Gesichter des Schweigens Die Systemische Mutism: Therapie/Symut als Therapie Alternative.* Idstein: Schutz-Kirchner.

Hartman, B. (2006) Gesichter des Schweigens. *Die Systemische Mutismus-Therapie/SYMUT als Therapiealternative.* Idstein: Schutz-Kirchner.

Hartshorn, M. (2006) *The Cost to the Nation of Children's Poor Communication.* London: ICAN.

Hayden, T.L. (1980) 'Classification of elective mutism.' *Journal of the American Academy of Child Psychiatry 19*, 118–133.

HM Government (1989) *The Children Act.* London: HMSO.

HM Government (2010) *The Equality Act.* London: HMSO.

Herbert, M. (1959) *Behaviour Modification Training Manual for School of Social Work.* Leicester: University of Leicester.

Hilari, H. and Botting, N. (2011) *The Impact of Communication Disability Across the Lifespan.* San Francisco, CA: J&R Press.

Hilbert, M. (2012) 'Towards a synthesis of cognitive biases: how information processing can bias decision making.' *Psychological Bulletin 138*, 2 , 211–237.

Irwin, J.R., Carter, A.S. and Briggs-Gowan, M.J. (2002) 'The social-emotional development of "late-talking" toddlers.' *Journal of the American Academy of Child and Adolescent Psychiatry 41*, 11, 1324–1331.

Johnson, M. and Jones, M. (2011) 'Silent Types.' *Nursery World 12-25*, 24–25.

Johnson, M. and Jones, M. (2012) *Supporting Quiet Children.* Cambridge: Lawrence Education.

Johnson, M. and Wintgens, A. (2001) *The Selective Mutism Resource Manual.* Bicester: Speechmark.

Johnson, M. and Wintgens, A. (2012) *Can I tell you about Selective Mutism?* London: Jessica Kingsley Publishers.

Jones, K. (2012) 'How intense is this silence? Developing a theoretical framework for the use of psychodynamic music therapy in the treatment of Selective Mutism in children with English as an additional language: a heuristic case study.' *British Journal of Music Therapy 26*, 2, 15–28.

Kagan, J. (1997) 'Temperament and the reactions to unfamiliarity.' *Child Development 68*, 139–143.

Kagan, J., Reznick, J.S. and Snidman, N. (1987) 'The physiology and psychology of behavioural inhibition in children.' *Child Development 58*, 1459–1473.

Kagan, J. and Snidman, N. (2004) *The Long Shadow of Temperament.* Cambridge, MA: Harvard University Press.

Kanehara, Y., Ayukawa, J., Sakamoto, K., Fukami, N. and Kitani, H. (2009) 'My experiences: 23 cases of elective mutism.' *The Journal of Ambulatory and General Paediatrics 12*, 1, 83–86.

Katz-Bernstein, N. (2003) *Aufbau der Sprach- und Kommunikationsfähigkeit bei redeflussgestörten Kindern. Ein sprachtherapeutisches Übungskonzept (8th edition).* Luzern: Edition SZH.

Katz-Bernstein, N. (2013) *Selective Mutism in Children. Manifestations, Diagnosis, Therapy (3rd edition).* Munich: Reinhardt.

Kawai, L. and Kawai, E. (1994) *Psychology and Guidance of Children with Selective Mutism.* Tokyo: Taken Publishing.

Kearney, C.C. (2010) *Helping Children with Selective Mutism and Their Parents: A Guide for School-Based Professionals.* Oxford: Oxford University Press.

Keen, D.V., Fonseca, S. and Wintgens, A. (2008) 'Selective mutism: A consensus based care pathway of good practice.' *Archives of Disease in Childhood 93*, 10, 838–844. Published online. Available at http://adc.bmj.com/content/93/10.toc, accessed on 25 April 2014.

Kelman, E. and Nicholas, A. (2008) *Practical Intervention for Early Childhood Stammering: Palin PCI Approach.* Milton Keynes: Speechmark.

Klein, R. (2009) 'Anxiety disorders.' *Journal of Child Psychology and Psychiatry 50*, 1–2, 153–162.

Klein, E.R., Armstrong, S.L. and Shipon-Blum, E. (2012) 'Assessing spoken language competence in children with selective mutism: using parents as test presenters.' *Communication Disorders Quarterly 20*, 10, 1–12.

Kolvin, I. and Fundudis, T. (1981) 'Elective mute children: psychological development and background factors.' *Journal of Child Psychology and Psychiatry 22*, 3, 219–232.

Kopp, S. and Gilberg, C. (1997) Selective mutism, a population-based study: a research note. *Journal of Child Psychology and Psychiatry 38*, 2, 257–262.

Kramer, J. (2006) 'Vergleich des selectiven mutismus mit dem frühkindlichen autismus.' *LOGOS Interdisziplinär 14*, 280–281.

Kratochwill, T. (1981) *Selective Mutism: Implications for Research and Treatment.* Hillsdale, NJ: Lawrence Erlbaum.

Kristensen, H. (2000) 'Selective mutism and comorbidity with developmental disorder/delay, anxiety disorder, and elimination disorder.' *Journal of the American Academy of Child and Adolescent Psychiatry 39*, 2, 249–256.

Kristensen, H. and Torgersen, S. (2001) 'MCM1-11 personality traits and symptom traits in parents of children with selective mutism: a case-control study.' *Journal of Abnormal Psychology 1104*, 648–652.

Krohn, D.D., Weckstein, S.M. and Wright, H.L. (1992) 'A study of the effectiveness of a specific treatment for elective mutism.' *Journal of the American Academy of Child and Adolescent Psychiatry 31*, 4, 711–718.

Krysanski, V.L. (2003) 'A brief review of Selective Mutism literature.' *The Journal of Psychology 137*, 1, 29–40.

Kumpulainen, K., Rasanen, E., Raaska, H. and Somppi, V. (1998) 'Selective mutism among second-graders in elementary school.' *European Child and Adolescent Psychiatry 7*, 1, 24–29.

Kussmaul, A. (1877) *Die Stoerungen der Sprache (2nd edition).* (First edition: Disturbances of Linguistic Function. Basel: Benno Schwabe.

Laskey, B. (2011) *Parenting Intervention for Young Anxious Children.* Association for Child and Adolescent Mental Health Occasional Papers No. 30, 20–27. London: ACAMH.

Law, J. and Garret, Z. (2004) 'Speech and language therapy: its potential role in CAMHS.' *Child and Adolescent Mental Health 9*, 2, 50–55.

Law, J., Reilly, S. and Snow, P. (1013) 'Child speech language and communication need re-examined in a public health context: a new direction for the speech and language therapy profession.' *International Journal of Language and Communication Disorders 48*, 5, 486–496.

Lebowitz, E. and Omer, H. (2013) *Treating Childhood and Adolescent Anxiety: A Guide for Caregivers.* Chichester: Wiley.

Lebrun, Y. (1990) *Mutism.* London: Whurr (now Chichester: Wiley).

Leinonen, E., Letts, C. and Smith, B.R. (2000) *Children's Pragmatic Communication Difficulties.* London: Whurr (now Chichester: Wiley).

Looff, D.H. (1971) *Appalachia's Children: The Challenge of Mental Health.* Lexington, KY: University Press of Kentucky.

Lord, C., Rutter, M., DiLavore, P.C. and Risi, S. (2000) *Autism Diagnostic Observation Schedule.* Los Angeles, CA: Western Psychological Services.

Magagna, J. (ed.) (2012) *The Silent Child: Communication Without Words.* London: Karnac.

Mahns, W. (2003) 'Speaking Without Talking: 50 Analytical Music Therapy Sessions with a Boy with Selective Mutism.' In S. Hadley (ed.) *Psychodynamic Music Therapy Case Studies.* New Haven, CT: Barcelona Publishers.

Manassis, K. (2009) 'Silent suffering: understanding and treating children with selective mutism.' *Expert Reviews 9*, 2, 235–243.

Manassis, K. and Tannock, R. (2008) 'Comparing interventions for selective mutism: a pilot study.' *La Revue Canadienne de Psychiatrie 53*, 10, 700–703.

Manassis, K., Fung, D., Tannock, R., Sloman, L., Fiksenbaum, L. and McInnes, A. (2003) 'Characterizing selective mutism: is it more than social anxiety?' *Depression and Anxiety 18*, 3, 153–161.

Manassis, K., Tannock, R., Garland, E.J., Minde, K., McInnes, A., and Clark, S. (2007) 'The sounds of silence: language, cognition and anxiety in selective mutism.' *Journal of the American Academy of Child and Adolescent Psychiatry* 46, 9, 1187–1195.

Markham, C. and Dean T. (2006) 'Research Report: Parents' and professionals' perceptions of quality of life in children with speech and language difficulty.' *International Journal of Language and Communication Disorders 41*, 2, 189–212.

Marks, I.M. (1969) *Fears and Phobias.* Oxford: Heinemann.

McHolm, A., Cunningham, C. and Vanier, M. (2005) *Helping Your Child with Selective Mutism: Practical Steps to Overcome a Fear of Speaking.* Oakland, CA: New Harbinger Publications.

McInnes, A., and Manassis, K. (2005) 'When silence is not golden: an integrated approach to selective mutism.' *Seminars in Speech and Language 26*, 3, 201–210.

McInnes, A., Fung, D., Manassis, K., Fiksenbaum, L. and Tannock, R. (2004) 'Narrative skills in children with selective mutism: an exploratory study.' *American Journal of Speech-Language Pathology 13*, 4, 304–315.

McLaughlin, M.R. (2011) 'Speech and language delay in children.' *American Family Physician 83*, 10, 1183–1188.

McLeod, S. and McKinnon, D. (2007) 'Prevalence of communication disorders compared with other learning needs in 14,500 primary and secondary school students.' *International Journal of Language and Communication Disorders 42*, 81, 37–59.

McWilliams, B.J., Morris, H.L. and Shelton, R.L. (1990) *Cleft Palate Speech (2nd edition).* Philadelphia, PA: B.C. Decker.

Meadows, S. (1993) *The Child as Thinker: The Development and Acquisition of Cognition in Childhood.* London: Routledge.

Merry, R. (1998) *Successful Children, Successful Teaching.* Buckingham: Open University Press.

Millard, S., Nicholas, A. and Cook, F. (2008) 'Is parent-child interaction therapy effective in reducing stuttering?' *Journal of Speech, Language and Hearing Research 51*, 3, 636–650.

Miller, E. (2008) *The Girl who Spoke with Pictures: Autism through Art.* London: Jessica Kingsley Publishers.

Miller, S.D., Hubble, M. and Duncan, B. (2008) 'Supershrinks: what is the secret of their success?' *Psychotherapy in Australia 14*, 4, 14–22.

Ministry of Education, Culture, Sports, Science and Technology (Japan) (2012) *Survey of Children who Attend Regular Classes, Who May Need Special Educational Support for a Possible Developmental Disorder.* Tokyo: Author.

Murray, L., Pearson , J., Bergeron, C., Schofield, E., Royal-Lawson, M. and Cooper, P.J. (2008) 'Intergenerational transmission of social anxiety: the role of social referencing processes in infancy.' *Child Development 79*, 1049–1064. Cited in Laskey, B. (2011) *Parenting Intervention for Young Anxious Children.* Association for Child and Adolescent Mental Health Occasional Papers No. 30, 20–27. London: ACAMH.

Myers, J., Willise, J. and Villalba, J. (2011) 'Promoting self-esteem in adolescents: the influence of wellness factors.' *Journal of Counseling and Development 89*, 1, 28–30.

Nind, M. and Hewett, D. (1994/1996/2001) *A Practical Guide to Intensive Interaction.* Birmingham: British Institute of Learning Disability (BILD).

Oerbeck, B., Stein, M.B., Wentzel-Larsen, T., Langsrud, O. and Kristensen, H. (2013) 'A randomized controlled trial of a home and school-based intervention for selective mutism – defocused communication and behavioural techniques.' *Child and Adolescent Mental Health.* Published online. doi:10.1111/camh.12045.

Omdal, H. (2007) 'Can adults who have recovered from selective mutism in childhood and adolescence tell us anything about the nature of the condition and/or recovery from it?' *European Journal of Special Needs Education 22*, 3, 237–253.

Omdal, H. and Galloway, D. (2007) 'Interviews with selectively mute children.' *Emotional and Behavioural Difficulties 12*, 3, 205–214.

Omdal, H. and Galloway, D. (2008) 'Could selective mutism be re-conceptualised as a specific phobia of expressive speech?' *Child and Adolescent Mental Health 13*, 2, 74–81.

Pellegrini, A.D. (2009) *The Oxford Handbook of the Development of Play.* Oxford: Oxford University Press.

Perednik, R. (2013) *The Selective Mutism Treatment Guide.* Jerusalem: Oaklands Press.

Preston-Dunlop, V. (1998) *Rudolf Laban: An Extraordinary Life.* London: Dance Books.

Prevezer, W. (1990) 'Music Interaction: Strategies for Tuning in to Autism.' In L. Mahon (ed.) *The Handbook of Play Therapy.* London: Routledge.

Rapee, R.M., Wignall, A., Spence, S.H., Cobham, V. and Lyneham, H. (2008) *Helping your Anxious Child: A Step-by-Step Guide for Parents (2nd edition).* Oakland, CA: New Harbinger.

RDF Media (2006) *Help Me to Speak: Part 2 – Selective Mutism.* Channel 4 Documentary.

Reed, C.F. (1963) 'Elective mutism in children: a reappraisal.' *Journal of Child Psychology and Psychiatry 4*, 2 , 99–107.

Reid, J.B., Hawkins, N., Keutzer, C., McNeal, S.A., Phelps, R.E. and Mees, H.L. (1967) 'A marathon behaviour modification of a selectively mute child.' *Journal of Child Psychology and Psychiatry 8*, 1, 27–30.

Robinson, J. and Burges, B. (2001) 'Joanne and Michele's Story: Working with John.' In T. O'Brian and P. Garner (eds) *Untold Stories: Learning Support Assistants and their Work*. Stoke on Trent, UK, and Sterling, USA: Trantham.

Roe, V. (1993) 'An interactive therapy group.' *Child Language, Teaching and Therapy* 9, 2, 133–140.

Roe, V. (2004) 'Interactive therapy in a school setting.' in Sage, R. and Sluckin, A. *Silent Children: Approaches to Selective Mutism*. Leicester: University of Leicester, 37–42.

Roe, V. (2011) *Silent Voices: Listening to Young People with Selective Mutism*. Leeds: British Education Index. Available at www.leeds.ac.uk/educol/documents/203095.pdf, accessed on 25 April 2014.

Roe, V. and Sluckin, A. (2014) 'The silent children.' *NASEN Special Magazine* 24–5, March.

Rogers, C. (1961) *On Becoming a Person: A Therapist's View of Psychotherapy*. London: Constable.

Royal College of Speech and Language Therapists (2006) 'Selective Mutism.' In *Communicating Quality 3: RCSLT's Guidance on Best Practice in Service Organization and Provision*. London: Author. Available at www.rcslt.org/speech_and_language_therapy/standards/CQ3_pdf, accessed on 16 July 2014.

Rutter, M. (2008) 'Diagnostic Concepts and Risk Processes.' In C.F. Norbury, J.B. Tomblin and D.V.M. Bishop (eds) *Understanding Developmental Language Disorders: From Theory to Practice*. Hove and New York, NY: Psychology Press.

Rutter, M., LeCouteur, A., and Lord, C. (2003) *ADI-R: The Autism Diagnostic Interview – Revised*. Los Angeles, CA: Western Psychological Services.

Sage, R. (2000) *Class Talk*. Stafford: Network Educational Press (now Bloomsbury).

Sage, R. (2003) *Lend Us Your Ears*. Stafford: Network Educational Press (now Bloomsbury).

Sage, R. (2004) 'The Communication Opportunity Group Scheme.' In R. Sage and A. Sluckin (eds) *Silent Children: Approaches to Selective Mutism*. Leicester: University of Leicester.

Sage, R. (2007) *Inclusion in Schools*. Stafford: Network Educational Press (now Bloomsbury).

Sage, R. (2011) *A Communicative Model for Developing Key Competencies in Senior School Students. A European Study of Inter-competency and Dialogue through Literature (IDIAL) – A Comenius Programme, 2009–11*. Final Report. Sofia, Bulgaria: ICCF.

Sage, R. (2012) 'Communication over curriculum? Comparing British and Japanese early years education.' *Education Today, Journal of the College of Teachers 62, 4*.

Sage, R. and Sluckin, A. (2004) *Silent Children: Approaches to Selective Mutism*. Leicester: University of Leicester.

Schopler, E. (1997) 'Implementation of TEACCH Philosophy.' In D.J. Cohen and
    F.R. Volkmar (eds) *Handbook of Autism and Pervasive Developmental Disorders.*
    New York, NY: Wiley.

Schwartz, R.H., Freedy, A.S. and Sheridan, M.J. (2006) 'Selective mutism: are
    primary care physicians missing the silence?' *Clinical Paediatrics 45*, 1, 43–48.

Serry, T., Rose, M. and Liamputtong, P. (2008) 'Oral language predictors for the
    at-risk reader: a review.' *International Journal of Speech-Language Pathology 10*,
    6, 392–403.

Sharkey, L. and McNicholas, F. (2012) 'Selective mutism: a prevalence study of
    primary school children in the Republic of Ireland.' Brief report. *Irish Journal
    of Psychiatric Medicine 29*, 1, 36–40.

Shaw, W.H. (1971) 'Aversive control in the treatment of elective mutism.' *Journal of
    the American Academy of Child Psychiatry 10*, 3, 572–581.

Sluckin, A. (1977) 'Children who do not talk at school.' *Child: Care, Health and
    Development 3*, 2, 69–79.

Sluckin, A. (2000) 'Selective mutism.' In J. Law, A. Parkinson and R. Tamhne (eds)
    Communication Difficulties in Childhood. London: Radcliffe Medical Press.

Sluckin, A. (2006a) 'Introducing and evaluating the video: "Silent Children –
    Approaches to Selective Mutism."' *SEBADA News 11*, 6, 22.

Sluckin, A. (2006b) 'Helping Selectively Mute Children at School.' In M. Hunter-
    Carsh, Y. Tiknar, P. Cooper and R. Sage (eds) *The Handbook of Social,
    Emotional and Behavioral Difficulties.* London and New York, NY: Continuum.

Sluckin, A. (2011) 'Supporting children with selective mutism.' *British Journal of
    School Nursing 6*, 7, 342–344.

Sluckin, A. and Jehu, D. (1969) 'A behavioural approach in the treatment of elective
    mutism.' *British Journal of Psychiatric Social Work 10*, 2, 70–73.

Sluckin, A. and Whittington, L. (2009) 'The Role of Charities in Supporting
    Diversity and Inclusion: the Selective Mutism Information & Research
    Association (SMIRA).' In R. Sage (ed.) *Meeting the Needs of Students with
    Diverse Backgrounds.* London: Continuum.

Sluckin, A., Foreman, N. and Herbert, M. (1991) 'Behavioural treatment programs
    and selectivity of speaking at follow-up in a sample of 25 selective mutes.'
    Australian Psychologist 26, 2, 132–137.

Smayling, J.M. (1959) 'Analysis of six cases of voluntary mutism.' *Journal of Speech
    and Hearing Disorders 24*, 1, 55–58.

Smit, A.B. and Hand, L. (1997) *The Smit-Hand Articulation and Phonology
    Evaluation.* Los Angeles, CA: Western Psychological Services.

Smith, B.R. (2004) 'What has Speech and Language Therapy to Offer to Selective
    Mutism?' In R. Sage and A. Sluckin (eds) *Silent Children – Approaches to
    Selective Mutism.* Leicester: University of Leicester.

Smith, B.R. and Leinonen, E. (1992) *Clinical Pragmatics; Unravelling the
    Complexities of Communicative Failure.* London: Chapman and Hall (later
    Stanley Thorne).

Smith, G.C. (2009) 'From consultation-liaison psychiatry to integrated care for multiple and complex needs.' *Australian and New Zealand Journal of Psychiatry* 43, 1, 1–12.

Steinhausen, H.C. and Juzi, C. (1996) 'Elective mutism: an analysis of 100 cases.' *Journal of the American Academy of Child and Adolescent Psychiatry 35*, 5, 606–614.

Steinhausen, H.C., Wachter, M., Laimbock, K. and Metzke, C.W. (2006) 'A long-term outcome study of selective mutisim in childhood.' *Journal of Child Psychology and Psychiatry 47*, 7, 751–756.

Stern, D.N. (2002) *The First Relationship: Infant and Mother.* Cambridge, MA: Harvard University Press. (Original work published 1977.)

Subellok, K., Katz-Bernstein, N., Bahrfeck-Wichitill, K. and Starke, A. (2012) 'DortMuT (Dortmunder Mutismus-Therapie): Eine sprachtherapeutische Konzeption für Kinder und Jugendliche mit selektivem Mutismus.' *LOGOS Interdisziplinär 20*, 2, 84–96.

Sweeney, M., Levitt, J., Westerholm, R., Gaskins, C. and Lipinski, C. (2013) 'Psychosocial Treatment of Anxiety Disorders Across the Lifespan.' In S.M. Stahl and B.A. Moore (eds) *Anxiety Disorders: A Guide for Integrating Psychopharmacology and Psychotherapy.* New York and London: Routledge.

Sylva, K. and Lunt, I. (1982) *Child Development: A First Course.* Oxford: Blackwell.

Taylor, G. (1997) 'Community building in schools: developing a Circle of Friends.' *Educational and Child Psychology 14*, 3.

Thirlwall, K., Cooper, P.J., Karalus, J., Voysey, M., Willetts, L. and Creswell, C. (2013) 'Treatment of child anxiety disorders via guided parent-delivered cognitive-behavioural therapy: randomised controlled trial.' *British Journal of Psychiatry 203*, 436-444.

Times, The (2012) 'Elizabeth Manners'. 8 June, p.55.

Timko, A., England, E., Herbert, J. and Foreman, E. (2010) 'The Implicit Relational Assessment Procedure as a measure of self-esteem.' *The Psychological Record 60*, 4, 679.

Tittnich, E. (1990) 'Clinical illustration: elective mutism.' *Journal of Children in Contemporary Society 21*, 1–2, 151–158.

Toppelberg, C.O., Tabors, P., Coggins, A., Lum, K. and Burger, C. (2005) 'Differential diagnosis of selective mutism in bilingual children.' *Journal of the American Academy of Child and Adolescent Psychiatry 44*, 6, 592–595.

Tough, J. (1976) *Listening to Children Talking: Skills in Early Childhood.* Schools Council Communication. London: Wardlock Drake Educational Associates.

Tramer, M. (1934) 'Electiver Mutismus bei Kindern.' *Z. Kinderpsychiat. 1*, 3035. (Translated by Anja Boeing.)

United Nations (1989) *Convention on the Rights of the Child: Fact Sheet 10.* Geneva: Centre for Human Rights.

Vecchio, J. and Kearney, C.A. (2005) 'Selective mutism in children: comparison to youths with and without anxiety disorders.' *Journal of Psychopathology and Behavioural Assessment 271*, 1, 31–37.

Vostanis, P., Humphrey, N., Fitzgerald, N., Deighton, J. and Volpert, M. (2013) 'How do schools promote emotional wellbeing among their pupils? Findings from a national scoping survey of mental health provision in English schools.' *Child and Adolescent Mental Health 18*, 3, 151–157.

Viana, A.G., Beidel, D.C. and Rabian, B. (2009) 'Selective mutism: a review and integration of the last 15 years.' *Clinical Psychology Review 29*, 57–67.

Vygotsky, L.S. (1978) *Mind and Society: The Development of Higher Psychological Processes.* Cambridge, MA: Harvard University Press.

Wallace, M. (1986) *The Silent Twins.* London: Baldwin.

Watson A.C.H. (2001) 'Embryology, Aetiology and Incidence.' In A.C.H. Watson, D.A. Sell and P. Grunwell (eds) *Management of Cleft Lip and Palate.* London: Whurr.

Weare, K. (2013) 'Child and adolescent mental health in schools.' *Child and Adolescent Mental Health 18*, 3, 129–130.

Welton, J. (2004) *Can I tell you about Asperger's Syndrome?* London: Jessica Kingsley Publishers.

Wiesmer, G. (2007) *Motor Speech Disorders.* Oxford: Plural.

Wilkins, R. (1985) 'A comparison of elective mutism and emotional disorders in children.' *British Journal of Psychiatry 146*, 2, 198–203.

Wong, P. (2010) 'Selective mutism: a review of etiology, comorbidities and treatment.' *Psychiatry 7*, 3, 23–31.

Wood, D. (1999) *How Children Think and Learn.* Oxford: Blackwell.

Wood, J.J., McLeod, B.D., Sigman, M., Hwang, W.C. and Chu, B.C. (2003) 'Parenting and childhood anxiety: theory, empirical findings, and future directions.' *Journal of Child Psychology and Psychiatry 44*, 1, 134–151.

World Health Organization (1994) *ICD 10.* Geneva: WHO.

Wright, H.L. (1968) 'A clinical study of children who refuse to talk in school.' *Journal of the American Academy of Child Psychiatry 7*, 4, 603–617.

Wright, H.H., Miller, M.D., Cook, M.A. and Littmann, J.R. (1985) 'Early identification and intervention with children who refuse to speak.' *Journal of the American Academy of Child and Adolescent Psychiatry 24*, 6, 739–746.

Wulbert, M., Nyman, B.A., Snow, D. and Owen, Y. (1973) 'The efficacy of stimulus fading and contingency management in the treatment of elective mutism.' *Journal of Applied Behavioral Analysis 6*, 435–444.

Yeganeh, R.M.A., Beidel, D.C., Turner, S.M., Armanndo, A.M.S. and Silverman, W.K. (2003) 'Clinical distinctions between Selective Mutism and social phobia: an investigation of childhood psychopathology.' *Journal of the American Academy of Child and Adolescent Psychiatry 42*, 9, 1069–1075.

Resources

SM organizations and support groups worldwide

A list of SM support organizations held by SMIRA is provided here for general information. Please note that SMIRA does not endorse and is not responsible for the advice or information given by any other organization or the content or conduct of any other website. The organizations are grouped here by language rather than by country.

ENGLISH

Selective Mutism Information & Research Association (SMIRA UK)
Registered Charity No. 1022673
Phone: 0800 2289765
www.smira.org.uk
E-mail: info@smira.co.uk
Facebook: Smira

Scottish SM Group
Facebook: Scottish Selective Mutism Group (SSMG)

ISPEAK (for SM adults)
www.ispeak.org.uk
E-Mail: carl@ispeak.org.uk

SMG-CAN (Canada)
www.selectivemutism.org
Facebook: The Selective Mutism Group

SM Foundation (USA)
www.selectivemutismfoundation.org
Facebook: The Selective Mutism Foundation

Carolyn Miller
The Selective Mutism Foundation, Inc.
P.O. Box 13133
SISSONVILLE
WV 25360-0133
USA

Sue Newman
The Selective Mutism Foundation, Inc.
P.O. Box 25972
Tamarac
FL 33320
USA

Selective Mutism Clinic
Suite 301, Level 3, 118 Christie Street
St Leonards
NSW 2065
Australia
Phone: 0405 430 530
www.selectivemutism.com.au

FRENCH
Ouvrir La Voix (OLV)
www.ouvrirlavoix.sitego.fr
Facebook: Ouvrir la Voix

ITALIAN
AIMuSe
www.aimuse.it
Facebook: AIMUSE

CHINESE
Taipei/HongKong
Facebook: www.facebook.com/groups/201513733329226

GERMAN
Mutismus Selbsthilfe Deutschland e.V.
www.mutismus.de

IG Mutismus Schweiz
www.mutismus.ch

SPANISH
Mutismo Selectivo – Argentina
Facebook: Mutismo Selectivo Argentina

POLISH
MUTYZM
www.mutyzmwybiorczy.pl
Facebook: MUTYZM

JAPANESE
Kanmoku Net
www.kanmoku.org
Facebook かんもくネット

VLAAMS/FLEMISH
Selectief Mutisme Vlaanderen
Facebook: Selectief Mutisme Vlaanderen

Other relevant associations and support groups
UK
Anxiety UK
www.anxietyuk.org.uk

British Association of Behavioural and Cognitive Psychotherapies (BABCP)
Imperial House
Hornby Street
Bury
Lancashire
BL9 5BN
Phone: 0161 705 4304
www.babcp.com

Fear Fighter
www.fearfighter.com

MIND The National Association for Mental Health
Mind Infoline: 0300 123 3393
E-mail: info@mind.org.uk
Legal Advice Line: 0300 466 6463
E-mail: legal@mind.org.uk
www.mind.org.uk

Following the links 'Information and support' / 'Tips for everyday living' / 'Wellbeing' can be helpful.

RALLI (Raising Awareness of Language Learning Impairments)
www.youtube.com/rallicampaign

See also: the UK government and educational websites mentioned in Chapter 15 of this volume.

AUSTRALIA
Anxiety Disorders Association
Victoria (ADAVIC)
P.O. Box 625
Kew
Victoria 3101

Social Anxiety Australia (SAA)
P.O. Box 94
Indooroopilly
Queensland

Speech Pathology Australia
Level 2/11–19 Bank Place
Melbourne
Victoria 3000
Phone: 03 9642 4899
www.speechpathologyaustralia.org.au

Triumph Over Phobia (TOP, NSW)
PO Box 213 Rockdale NSW

NEW ZEALAND
Social Anxiety Support Group
Floor 2
Securities House
221 Gloucester Street
P.O. Box 13167
Christchurch

USA
Anxiety and Depression Association of America (ADDAA)
www.adaa.org

The Association for (previously the Advancement of)
Behavioral and Cognitive Therapies (ABCT)
305 7th Avenue
16th Floor
New York
NY 10001
www.abct.org

Institute for Behavior Therapy
20 East 49th Street
2nd Floor
New York
NY 10017
www.ifbt.com

Smart Center
505 N. Old York Road
Jenkintown Square – Lower Level
Jenkintown,
PA 19046
Phone: 215 887 5748
www.selectivemutismcenter.org

American Speech–Language–Hearing Association
2200 Research Boulevard,
Rockville, MD 20850-3289.
Phone: 301 296 5650.
www.asha.org/public/speech/disorders/selectivemutism

Apps

Headspace (mindfulness techniques) for Apple, IOS and Android

Way of Life (allows and encourages monitoring of progress toward goals) for IOS

Mindshift (strategies for anxiety) for Apple, IOS and Android

Published materials

Silent Children: Approaches to Selective Mutism (DVD, 2004), available, together
with or separately from the book of the same name by Rosemary Sage and
Alice Sluckin, from Lindsay Whittington, SMIRA Co-ordinator, 5 Keyham
Close, Humberstone, Leicester, LE5 1FW, UK.

Collins-Donnelly, K. (2012) *Starving the Anger Gremlin*. London: Jessica Kingsley Publishers.

Whitson, S. (2011) *How to be Angry: An Assertive Anger Expression Guide for Kids and Teens*. London: Jessica Kingsley Publishers.

Cartwight-Hatton, S., Lasky, B., Rust, S. and McNally, D. (2010) *From Timid to Tiger: A Treatment Manual for Parenting the Anxious Child*. Chichester: Wiley.

Chansky, Tamar E. (2014) *Freeing Your Child from Anxiety (2nd edition)*. New York, NY: Harmony Books/Random House.

Creswell, C. and Willetts, L. (2007) *Overcoming Your Child's Fears and Worries: A Self-Help Guide Using Cognitive Behavioral Techniques*. London: Robinson.

Heubner, D. (2005) *What to Do When You Worry Too Much: A Kid's Guide to Overcoming Anxiety*. Washington DC: APA/Magination Press.

Heubner, D (2007) *What to Do When Your Brain Gets Stuck: A Kid's Guide to Overcoming OCD*. Washington DC: APA/Magination Press.

Courses
CLASS training in Selective Mutism
University College London (UCL)
www.ucl.ac.uk/psychlangsci/students/professional/class

Relaxation for Living
29 Burwood Park Road
Walton on Thames
Surrey
KT12 5LH

Floor-time play therapy
www.selectivemutism.org

Courses on confidence-building
www.collegeofteachers.ac.uk/Learn

UK Helplines
Afasic (Association for All Speech Impaired Children)
0845 3 55 55 77 or 020 77490 9410

Anxiety UK
08444 775 774

No Panic
0800 138 8889
01952 680460

Suppliers

These companies produce helpful 'talking' (i.e. recordable) photograph albums and a variety of small recordable message devices that can easily be carried by children.

Living made easy for children

www.livingmadeeasy.org.uk/children/hand-held-communication-aids-_-direct-selection-p/chatterbox-10-0110792-1415-information.htm

Inclusive Technology

www.inclusive.co.uk

Special Direct

www.specialdirect.com

Taskmaster

www.taskmasteronline.co.uk

Miscellaneous

Silent Voices © Victoria Roe 2011

jvjr1@alumni.leicester.ac.uk

The Virtual Issue (Child and adolescent mental health in schools, September 2013)
Free access resource. http://onlinelibrary.wiley.com/
store/10.1111/(ISSN)1475-3588/asset/homepages/Editorial_
for_CAMH_in_schools_VI_final.pdf?v=1&s=6050a32b1ee
3bc478d9dc79312964d2789010bcb&isAguDoi=false

Contributors

Dr David Bramble is a Consultant Child and Adolescent Learning Disability Psychiatrist working for Shropshire Community Health Services NHS Trust in a specialist CAMHS-Learning Disability team.

Hilary Cleator is a Specialist Speech Pathologist and researcher currently working in Australia.

Dr Tony Cline is Co-Director of the CPD Doctorate in Educational Psychology, University College London, and Emeritus Professor at the University of Bedford. His research interests include the education of bilingual and trilingual children, selective mutism, literacy learning difficulties of bilingual pupils, the education of minority ethnic children in mainly white schools and child language brokering at school.

Charlotte Firth is a Speech and Language Therapist – Advanced Level, Scarborough area SLT Department, York Teaching Hospital NHS Foundation Trust.

Geoffrey Gibson is a Lecturer in English as a Foreign Language at the University of Hull, and Director of Studies for the School of Languages, Linguistics, and Culture.

Miriam Jemmett is a Highly Specialist Speech and Language Therapist working across primary and secondary schools for East Kent Hospitals University NHS Foundation Trust.

Maggie Johnson is Principal Speech and Language Therapist for Selective Mutism, Kent Community Health NHS Trust.

Sue Johnson is a SENCO working in Leicestershire.

Catherine Jones is a Music Therapist and Researcher working for Music Therapy Lambeth, which is a non-profit organization.

Jane Kay is Targeted Support Youth Advisor, Youth and Family Support Service, Children, Family and Adult Services, East Riding of Yorkshire Council.

Keiko Kakuta is a Specialist Paediatric Clinical Psychologist at Sanda Municipal Hospital, Hyogo prefecture. She also works as a school counsellor for primary school and high school.

Professor Dr Nitza Katz-Bernstein is a Consultant, Supervisor, Child and Adolescent Psychotherapist and Speech Therapist. At present (since retirement 2008) she is a visiting Professor at the Tel-Aviv University, Department of Communication Disorders, and at the Krems-Donau University in Austria.

Denise Lanes is a Retired Specialist Teacher.

Jenny Packer is a Specialist Speech and Language Therapist.

Victoria Roe is Deputy Chair of SMIRA, the UK Selective Mutism Information & Research Association. She is a retired teacher and former SENCO.

Professor Rosemary Sage is a Speech and Language Therapist, psychologist and teacher. She has latterly been a professor in communication in Liverpool and visiting professor in Japan and Cuba. She is presently Professor of Education and Dean of Academic Studies at the College of Teachers, in the London Institute of Education.

Jyoti Sharma is a Play Interaction Specialist (Instructor – unqualified Teacher) and Autism Outreach worker for Leicester City Council.

Alice Sluckin, OBE, is a retired Senior Psychiatric Social Worker and Chair of SMIRA. Over a long career she has published on various topics, notably maternal bonding, as well as selective mutism.

Benita Rae Smith is a retired Speech and Language Therapist and retired Senior Lecturer in Speech Pathology and Therapy. She has co-authored several works on the practical applications of pragmatics theory.

Dr Carl Sutton is a Software Engineer currently studying psychology. He maintains and co-ordinates ispeak, the support network for adults and teenagers with Selective Mutism.

Lindsay Whittington is Co-ordinator of SMIRA.

Alison Wintgens is a retired Specialist Speech and Language Therapist.

Subject Index

Author Index

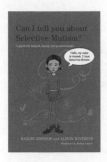

Can I tell you about Selective Mutism?
A guide for friends, family and professionals
Maggie Johnson and Alison Wintgens
Illustrated by Robyn Gallow
Paperback: £8.99 / $13.95
ISBN: 978 1 84905 289 4
56 pages

Meet Hannah – a young girl with Selective Mutism (SM). Hannah invites readers to learn about SM from her perspective, helping them to understand what it is, what it feels like to have SM, and how they can help.

This illustrated book is packed with accessible information and will be an ideal introduction to SM. It shows family, friends and teachers how they can support a child with the condition and is also a good place to start when encouraging children with SM to talk about how it affects them.

Contents: Acknowledgements. Introduction. 1. Introducing Hannah who has Selective Mutism. 2. Tension, panic and phobia. 3. Speaking freely at home. 4. It's not refusal to speak. 5. Playing with other children. 6. Talking in the classroom. 7. Feeling stressed and frustrated. 8. Speaking with the wider family. 9. Associated fears or phobias. 11. Telling the class about Selective Mutism. 12. How other children can help. 13. How teachers can help. 14. How parents can help. Recommended reading, DVDs, websites and organisations.

Maggie Johnson is a speech and language therapist and educational consultant specialising in childhood communication disorders and Selective Mutism (SM). With thirty years' experience in education and community settings, Maggie works closely with families and schools in East Kent and provides training and workshops for schools, parents and health professionals across the UK and abroad. She lives in Ramsgate, UK. **Alison Wintgens** was a consultant speech and language therapist in child and adolescent mental health based at St George's Hospital until her retirement in July 2011. She has worked for over 20 years with children who have SM and lives in London. Now she continues to write and teach, and is the advisor on SM to the Royal College of Speech and Language Therapists. Maggie and Alison have both published extensively in the field of speech and language therapy and are advisors to the Selective Mutism Information & Research Association (SMIRA). **Robyn Gallow's** illustrations have been used in a number of educational titles. She lives in London, and is involved in both fashion and illustrating.

Also available in the **Can I tell you about…** series

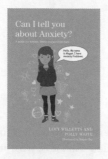

Can I tell you about Anxiety?
A guide for friends, family and professionals
Lucy Willetts and Polly Waite
Illustrated by Kaiyee Tay
Paperback: £8.99 / $14.95
ISBN: 978 1 84905 527 7
56 pages

Meet Megan – a young girl who has an anxiety disorder. Megan invites readers to learn about anxiety from her perspective, helping them to understand why she sometimes feels anxious and how this affects her thoughts, feelings and behaviours. Megan talks about techniques she has learnt to help manage her anxiety, and how people around her can help.

With illustrations throughout, this will be an ideal way to explore anxiety difficulties. It shows family, friends and teachers how they can support someone who experiences anxiety and will be an excellent way to start a conversation about anxiety, in the classroom or at home. Suitable for readers aged 7 upwards.

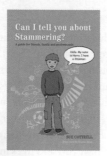

Can I tell you about Stammering?
A guide for friends, family and professionals
Sue Cottrell
Illustrated by Sophie Khan
Paperback: £8.99 / $13.95
ISBN: 978 1 84905 415 7
56 pages

Meet Harry – a young boy who stammers. Harry invites readers to learn about what it is like to stammer from his perspective and how it affects his daily life and makes him feel. He talks about techniques that can help reduce stammering and describes how friends, family and others can help him to feel at ease and reduce his stammer further.

This illustrated book is full of useful information and will be an ideal introduction for young people, aged 7 upwards, as well as parents, friends, teachers and speech therapists working with children who stammer. It is also an excellent starting point for group discussions at home or school

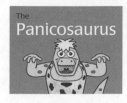

The Panicosaurus

Managing Anxiety in Children Including Those with Asperger Syndrome

K.I. Al-Ghani

Illustrated by Haitham Al-Ghani

Hardback: £12.99 / $19.95

ISBN: 978 1 84905 356 3

56 pages

Have you ever felt a sense of dread and worry creeping over you?

That might be the Panicosaurus coming out to play…

Sometimes the Panicosaurus tricks Mabel's brain into panicking about certain challenges, such as walking past a big dog on the street or when her favourite teacher is not at school. With the help of Smartosaurus, who lets her know there is really nothing to be afraid of, Mabel discovers different ways to manage Panicosaurus, and defeat the challenges he creates for her.

This fun, easy-to-read and fully illustrated storybook will inspire children who experience anxiety, and encourage them to banish their own Panicosauruses with help from Mabel's strategies. Parents and carers will like the helpful introduction, explaining anxiety in children, and the list of techniques for lessening anxiety at the end of the book.

K. I. Al-Ghani is a special educational needs teacher who has worked for more than 35 years in the field of education. She is currently a specialist teacher for inclusion support and is involved with training professionals, students and parents in aspects of ASD. As an author and a mother of a son with ASD – the illustrator Haitham Al-Ghani – she has spent the last 25 years researching the enigma that is autism. **Haitham Al-Ghani** is 27 years of age. He earned a triple distinction in multimedia studies and was the 2007 winner of the Vincent Lines Award for creative excellence. Haitham is an author, cartoon animator and the illustrator of many children's books.

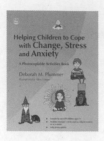

Helping Children to Cope with Change, Stress and Anxiety

A Photocopiable Activities Book

Deborah M. Plummer

Illustrated by Alice Harper

Paperback: £17.99/ $29.95

ISBN: 978 1 84310 960 0

144pp

Plummer offers over 100 activities aimed at helping children to build emotional resilience. With a mixture of short, snappy activities and longer guided visualizations, these exercises are suitable for use with individuals or groups, and many are appropriate for use with children with complex needs or speech and language difficulties.

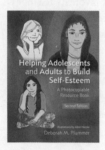

Helping Adolescents and Adults to Build Self-Esteem

A Photocopiable Resource Book

2nd edition

Deborah M. Plummer

Paperback: £25.00/ $39.95

ISBN: 978 1 84905 425 6

280pp

Brimming with innovative ideas for supporting the development of healthy self-esteem, this fully updated and expanded new edition of Deborah M. Plummer's popular resource is an indispensable aid to those working with adolescents and young adults. The easy-to-use photocopiable activity sheets are suitable for work with individuals and with groups.

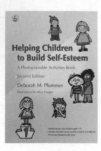

Helping Children to Build Self-Esteem

A Photocopiable Activities Book

2nd edition

Deborah M. Plummer

Illustrated by Alice Harper

Paperback: £19.99/ $32.95

ISBN: 978 1 84310 488 9

288pp

This activities book will support teaching staff, therapists and carers in encouraging feelings of competence and self-worth in children and their families. It is primarily designed for use with individuals and groups of children aged 7-11, but the ideas can easily be adapted for older and younger children and children with learning difficulties.